CRITICAL ISSUES in HEALTHCARE POLICY and POLITICS in the GULF COOPERATION COUNCIL STATES

CRITICAL ISSUES in HEALTHCARE POLICY and POLITICS in the GULF COOPERATION COUNCIL STATES

Ravinder Mamtani, MD
Albert B. Lowenfels, MD
Editors

جـامـعـة جـورجـتـاون قـطـر
GEORGETOWN UNIVERSITY QATAR

Center *for* International *and* Regional Studies

Published in Cooperation with the Center for International and Regional Studies, Georgetown University in Qatar

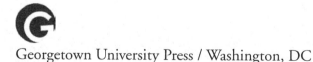

Georgetown University Press / Washington, DC

The publisher is not responsible for third-party websites or their content. URL links were active at time of publication.

Library of Congress Cataloging-in-Publication Data

Names: Mamtani, Ravinder, editor. | Lowenfels, Albert B., editor.
Title: Critical Issues in Healthcare Policy and Politics in the Gulf
    Cooperation Council States / Ravinder Mamtani and Albert B. Lowenfels,
    editors.
Description: Washington, DC : Georgetown University Press, 2017. | Includes
    bibliographical references and index. | Description based on print version
    record and CIP data provided by publisher; resource not viewed.
Identifiers: LCCN 2017008734 (print) | LCCN 2017011974 (ebook) | ISBN 9781626165007
    (hc : alk. paper) | ISBN 9781626165014 (pb : alk. paper) | ISBN 9781626165021 (eb)
Subjects: LCSH: Medical policy--Persian Gulf Region. | Medical care--Persian
    Gulf Region.
Classification: LCC RA395.P39 (ebook) | LCC RA395.P39 C75 2017 (print) | DDC
    362.10953--dc23
LC record available at https://lccn.loc.gov/2017008734

18 17   9 8 7 6 5 4 3 2 First printing

Printed in the United States of America

Cover design by 4eyesdesign
Cover images by iStock (Cleveland Clinic in Abu Dhabi by typhoonski) and
Shutterstock (Arabic door by kaitshot)

CONTENTS

FOREWORD

Although recent scholarship has drawn attention to educational developments in the Gulf Cooperation Council (GCC) states, similar contributions addressing health policy development and implementation in the region are largely lacking. Most recent work on healthcare systems in the Middle East, North Africa, and the Gulf countries consists of reports compiled by consulting firms such as Booz & Company, McKinsey & Company, and Alpen Capital. And though such reports focus on how existing healthcare structures can be transformed into modern healthcare systems, they lack academic rigor and tend to ignore larger, policy-related issues. As for the social scientists, there has been a striking dearth of contributions addressing policies and practices of healthcare systems of different states.

The *Eastern Mediterranean Health Journal*, the flagship health periodical of the World Health Organization, regularly publishes highly technical articles related to very specific case studies of a particular health-related issue in a subset of a population, including groups in Saudi Arabia. However, little has been published that addresses healthcare policy and politics from an academic perspective. A recent series in *The Lancet* titled "Health in the Arab World: A View from Within" (February 2014) provides a fairly comprehensive look at healthcare in the Arab world but does not present much data from the Gulf region. Similarly, *Public Health in the Arab World*—an edited volume published in 2012 by Cambridge University Press—focuses on the non-Gulf Arab countries. The present volume is unique in that it focuses exclusively on the states of the GCC and will contribute much-needed comprehensive analyses of healthcare policy and politics in these states.

This book emerged from two workshops organized by the Center for International and Regional Studies at Georgetown University in Qatar, and it represents a combined effort by the Qatar campuses of Georgetown's Walsh School of Foreign Service and Weill Cornell Medicine–Qatar. The collaborative effort involving all the contributors to this volume was enhanced by intensive consultations with other specialist colleagues to improve the focus and depth of the chapters' analyses. The result of this comprehensive collaboration is a volume in which each individual chapter presents a study that is an original work of scholarship making a significant contribution to the field.

This book provides a much-needed perspective on healthcare policy and politics in the GCC states, and contextualizes the efforts and the challenges they have encountered in modernizing their healthcare systems. It should be essential reading for academics, scholars, policymakers, and students interested in learning about the GCC states' current thinking on health policymaking, and the latest information on systemic efforts to transform health systems in the region. The book is also likely to appeal to practicing health professionals and other key actors in the healthcare sector in the GCC. Last but not least, this volume will be of interest to a large number of expatriates who are interested in the underlying themes that are shaping healthcare policy and practice within the region.

Javaid Sheikh, MD
Dean, Weill Cornell Medicine–Qatar
Doha

ACKNOWLEDGMENTS

Many people have generously contributed their time in the planning and preparation of this book. We are very grateful to all the authors for their contributions, cooperation, and responses to the editorial suggestions.

Our appreciation goes to many of our colleagues at Georgetown University in Qatar and Weill Cornell Medicine–Qatar who have helped with and guided many editing and administrative aspects in the assembly of our final manuscript. We would like to specifically thank Marco Ameduri, Raji Anand, Zahra Babar, Doris Lowenfels, Jaishree Mamtani, and Alan Weber. The editing and formatting assistance that was provided by Laura-Louise Fairley is also greatly appreciated.

Particular gratitude is owed to Mehran Kamrava, director of the Center for International and Regional Studies at Georgetown University in Qatar, who was the main force in conceptualizing the theme of this book, initiating discussions and workshops on its contents, and continuing to provide invaluable guidance at every stage of its evolution. The book would never have been written without his help.

Javaid Sheikh, MD, dean of Weill Cornell Medicine–Qatar, deserves our special thanks for his guidance and energetic support. As an experienced medical educator and a renowned healthcare executive, he was particularly helpful in ensuring that the contents of this book reflect a wide range of viewpoints.

Finally, we would like to express our sincere gratitude to the Qatar Foundation and its leadership for their invaluable, ongoing support in promoting an environment that encourages scholarly engagement in pivotal areas of health policy and regional development.

Ravinder Mamtani, MD
Albert B. Lowenfels, MD

INTRODUCTION

Ravinder Mamtani and Albert B. Lowenfels

About fifty million people live in the Gulf Cooperation Council (GCC) states of Bahrain, Kuwait, Oman, Qatar, Saudi Arabia, and the United Arab Emirates. The GCC's critical geographic location between Europe and Asia has resulted in an increase in both inhabitants and visitors, in what was once a relatively remote region. Geographically contiguous—and located just 25 degrees north of the equator—the region has a desert climate marked by excessive summer heat, minimal rainfall, and an increased likelihood of dust storms.[1] These geographic factors play a deterministic role in the overall health of the region's inhabitants.

Within the GCC, population and economic growth over the past several decades has been rapid, as has been the region's integration into the global economy.[2] These factors have led to a substantial increased demand for a modern, capable healthcare system to satisfy the needs of the population. This rapid, unprecedented demand for healthcare has resulted in the majority of services and professionals being sourced from outside the region. Before the unprecedented growth of the energy industry within the GCC, healthcare was limited to individuals mostly practicing traditional medicine, and to very small hospitals staffed by a handful of health professionals. If this level of healthcare had persisted, it would have severely limited regional growth (table I.1). Many of the healthcare workers in the GCC have been trained outside the region, emphasizing the need to increase training capacity for the nationals in each country.

Beginning at the end of the twentieth century and continuing until the present, the Gulf region's countries have devoted considerable efforts to boosting the healthcare sector. Although estimates vary greatly between different sources, healthcare-related costs are increasing rapidly, and are projected to reach $60 billion by 2025. Despite this considerable financial investment, the region still does not match other developed nations in infrastructure and capacity. Rapid changes to the environment and lifestyle of the Gulf region over the course of only a few decades have completely changed the region's health profile.

Table I.1 **Distribution of Health Professionals per 10,000 Population, 2014**

Country	Physicians	Dentists	Nurses
Bahrain	9	24	2.3
Kuwait	18	46	3.5
Oman	22	50	2.6
Qatar	77	119	5.8
Saudi Arabia	7.7	23	0.9
United Arab Emirates	19	41	4.3
United Kingdom	28	88	5.4
Norway	37	134	8.6

Source: World Health Organization, "World Health Statistics 2014."

Until now, healthcare costs for citizens of the GCC have been primarily borne by their respective governments, and this has become a major challenge for the state. Despite the availability of free medical care, many citizens of wealthier states, such as Qatar and the United Arab Emirates, prefer to receive medical treatment abroad instead of relying on the national healthcare system. In most cases the additional costs for overseas treatment are funded by the state, substantially increasing the burden of healthcare costs. Also, with rising healthcare costs, we see a shift across the region, from the traditional approach of publicly run healthcare to alternative models. Some of the Gulf states have been trying to make the healthcare sector more attractive for the private sector. It is assumed that if the region's governments, by providing infrastructure and a strengthened regulatory environment, create a more enabling environment, then the private sector can play a more active role in managing regional health-care needs. However, it is unclear whether the governments envision a complete departure from the current state-led healthcare system or if governments prefer a supportive role for the private sector while still retaining the core responsibility for healthcare provision.

In the Gulf states the healthcare field is currently dominated by expatriate ex-pertise. Public health professionals have drawn attention to the critical need for the GCC to develop national and regional expertise in healthcare management. Many regional states have recently established state-of-the-art medical teaching and training programs, specifically designed to build a national cadre of health professionals. Many would never have expected Cornell, an Ivy League univer-sity—ranked among the most prestigious in the world—to establish one of its core medical education programs on foreign soil. Now, however, Weill Cornell

Medicine–Qatar (WCM-Q) is Qatar's first medical school and is dedicated to excellence in education, patient care, research, and public health. A pioneer of coeducation at the university level, WCM-Q offers a fully integrated, six-year premedical and medical education program, leading to the awarding of Cornell University's doctor of medicine degree.

It is also essential to build national expertise in the management of health-care. Medical technology and population health remain key determinants of strong healthcare systems, so additional areas—such as research, information technology, and healthcare management—are pivotal to strengthen the new strategies developed by the states.

Major successes in combating infectious diseases and improving standards of primary healthcare have been reflected in key health indicators—such as the decreasing levels of infant and maternal mortality rates and dramatic increases in life expectancy. Life expectancy is a simple measure of improvement of the healthcare system over time. As a result of several factors, life expectancy improved in all the GCC states during the twenty-three-year period from 1990 to 2013, with an average gain of about four to eight years. Table I.2 summarizes recent basic health statistics for each of the six GCC states. The life expectancy in the GCC, as shown in table I.2, is comparable to those of other high-income countries.

As the overall health of the region's population has improved, new patterns and trends in healthcare have emerged that pose different and yet significant challenges. For example, diseases related to the lifestyle of wealthy countries, such as diabetes, hypertension, and heart disease—which were once rare—are now common. These new challenges require highly trained and expertly skilled healthcare workers; an environment that supports local training, state-of-the-art diagnostic laboratories, research production, and dissemination; and knowledge acquisition to meet emerging healthcare needs.

Managing the healthcare needs of the region also requires accurate, up-to-date statistics. Such information is not always available in the GCC, which limits the ability to allocate resources. Thus, though the industry is rapidly evolving, critical decision making pertaining to healthcare issues is hampered by the limited availability of information, which underscores the need for additional research in the area. This volume discusses critical, pressing healthcare politics and policy issues in the GCC states. Specifically, it examines the GCC's rapidly changing health profile, the existing conditions of its healthcare systems, and the challenges posed to healthcare management across its six countries.

Table I.2 **Demographics of the GCC States**

Country	Population (1,000s)	Median Age (years)	Population Growth Rate (%)	Life Expectancy (years)	< 5 mortality (per 1,000 live births)
Bahrain	1,332	30	1.1	77	6
Kuwait	3,369	29	3.6	78	10
Oman	3,632	26	5.8	76	11
Qatar	2,169	32	2.9	79	8
Saudi Arabia	28,829	28	2.1	76	16
United Arab Emirates	9,346	30	0.8	76	8

Sources: WHO Global Health Observatory, "Country Statistics," January 2015, http://www.who.int /gho/countries/en/; World Bank, "The World Bank Indicators: Population Growth," http://data .worldbank.org/indicator/SP.POP.GROW?view=chart.

ABOUT THIS VOLUME

This book begins with a historical overview of the development and transformation of healthcare in the Gulf region. In chapter 1 Nabil Kronfol reminds us that in the early part of the twentieth century, the most common diseases in the region were malaria, trachoma, intestinal parasites, malnutrition, and anemia; today, these diseases have disappeared, only to be replaced by what we now call "lifestyle diseases." Kronfol also points out how many of the region's healthcare needs in the early part of the twentieth century were supplied from existing sources in Europe and the United States, sometimes by religious organizations. In the absence of a reliable healthcare system, the best treatment option was to seek healthcare services in a non-GCC country. To a certain extent, native citizens and expatriates still seek medical treatment abroad, especially for more complicated conditions.

Kronfol points out that a critical advance for regional medical care was the development of medical schools. All the GCC states now have medical schools, often with a connection to a medical school in a non-GCC country. The establishment of WCM-Q, mentioned above, is a case in point. The expectation is that physicians trained in local and regional schools will eventually assume leadership roles and deliver healthcare to the GCC population.

In a discussion of regional goals and accomplishments, Kronfol emphasizes that most of the GCC states have signed the Declaration of Alma Ata to promote the health of all the world's people, under the auspices of the World Health Organization; and there are some areas of cooperation, such as the formation of the Secretariat of the Gulf Ministers of Health. Developing a regional certification mechanism and a unified research institution are areas where further cooperation could lead to mutual benefit for all the GCC states.

In chapter 2 Dionysis Markakis turns our attention to the politics of health-care in the region. He points out that in this region, healthcare is a major political issue because citizens, who are untaxed, benefit from the healthcare bestowed on them by monarchial governments. The investment is large and has increased steadily during the past few years. As in chapter 1, he notes that the present healthcare system is built on a foundation of healthcare introduced in the mid twentieth century from European and other foreign nations. Various GCC states are modernizing their healthcare systems with outside help from leading institutions such as Harvard University, Imperial College London, Johns Hopkins University, and WCM-Q. In addition to building training ca-pacity, hundreds of new hospital projects have been completed or are under way, with construction costs running to several billion dollars. With facilities located mainly in urban areas, healthcare is increasingly concentrated in cities, with special problems related to the growing epidemic of lifestyle diseases, such as obesity and diabetes.

Healthcare in all countries has a political dimension, but in the GCC states, in addition to race and gender, there is an additional dimension based on the highly desirable health benefits conferred by citizenship status. Accepting these benefits implies acceptance of the underlying political structure. Markakis points out that a strong healthcare system is one factor leading to political sta-bility. He reminds us about the unique nature of the financing of the health-care system; rather than being supported by taxation, as in most countries, oil revenue supports the considerable costs of healthcare. Where will the money to support healthcare come from once income from energy sources vanishes? A strong, effective healthcare system can lead to a new source of revenue from medical tourism, which is just in its infancy but has proved to be a stimulus for growth in other regions, such as Asia. All of the GCC states will need to address the issue of financial support for the health system.

The demographics of the region have a significant impact on the needs and conditions of the healthcare system. A division of the population into the cat-egories of nationals, highly skilled expatriates with greater disposable incomes, and the large numbers of low-income migrant workers creates different health profiles and needs for different segments of the populace.

A key element for a successful healthcare system is an adequate, well-trained, and well-motivated professional workforce. In chapter 3 Mohamad Alameddine and his coauthors discuss this issue by examining the entire GCC region and by also providing a state-specific analysis. As in the book's other chapters, the authors point out that the GCC's rapid population growth has resulted in a shortage of native-born healthcare workers, forcing each of the countries to rely heavily on individuals trained in other countries. In addition to an overall shortage of healthcare workers, the gender distribution is skewed, with females occupying positions in the lower-ranking healthcare labor force, though there are few females employed as physicians or dentists. This could be a potential problem—if, for example a female physician was not available for a female patient who prefers to be treated by a female rather than by a male physician.

Ratios of providers to population are low throughout the GCC, and the collaborative efforts of the GCC states with European and US medical schools will generate insufficient graduates to service the rapidly growing GCC population. For some countries, foreign-trained physicians account for 70 percent of the physician workforce. For the foreseeable future, foreign-trained healthcare workers will be required to supply the bulk of the region's needs. This brings up another set of problems, because the foreign workforce comes with different levels of training, different languages, and potential difficulties in communicating with patients.

There are also other healthcare issues, such as an oversupply of specialists and a limited supply of primary care or family physicians, a problem that is not unique to the GCC. Moreover, there are no region-specific guidelines for education or for judging standards of healthcare across the region. This deficiency leads many patients to opt for treatment outside rather than within the region.

Mental health is a major component of the global burden of disease. In chapter 4 Suhaila Ghuloum and Hassen Al-Amin provide an overview of the extent of mental illness and facilities available for its treatment in GCC states. All six GCC states have a mental health plan, but the degree of effort expended within each country necessary to achieve the stipulated goals varies. Based on limited information, the amount of spending on mental health is less than 5 percent of total healthcare expenditures.

One major roadblock to progress in supplying mental healthcare needs is a lack of information about the extent of the problem. This lack is compounded by the stigmatization of mental illness in Arab countries. Patients seek treatment only when symptoms are acute, and patients often discontinue therapy when they show signs of improvement. There is an additional issue because male migrant workers as a group face extremely stressful conditions, and they may be reluctant to report symptoms of mental illness because of a fear of losing their job.

As pointed out in chapter 3, on healthcare human resources, there is a shortage of adequately trained staff members to supply mental healthcare needs in all the GCC states. This means that patients will be treated by healthcare providers who lack the cultural sensitivity to deal with a difficult mental health crisis, and in many instances may not be fluent in Arabic. Most mental healthcare is concentrated in psychiatric hospitals, whereas, in other regions, the trend is to provide therapy in nonhospital settings.

Similar to issues related to mental health, substance abuse in the GCC states is also seldom discussed. In chapter 5 Samir Al-Adawi deals with this major global problem. The GCC states are near trade routes for the transporting of drugs from drug-producing nations, which could be a factor leading to an increase in the prevalence of substance abuse. Information about the extent of drug abuse is difficult to obtain because, as in many non-Arab countries, there is an ambivalent attitude about drug abuse. Are drug abusers individuals who have an illness, or are they criminals who should be prosecuted? Many regard drug abuse as a moral failure.

Information about the prevalence of drug abuse is obtained primarily from hospital sources rather than from community sources, leading to underestimates. Alcohol is banned completely or partially in all the GCC states, and therefore alcohol addiction is less common than in non-Arab countries. But because it is illegal, patients who are addicted to alcohol have difficulty obtaining treatment within the GCC, providing a reason for seeking treatment abroad. However, Al-Adawi reports that alcohol abuse exists as an unrecognized prob lem, even in countries such as Saudi Arabia, where it is totally banned.

Nicotine-related addiction from smoking tobacco leads to deleterious health effects and is common throughout the GCC states. Smoking is much more common in males, although water pipe smoking, which has similarly deleterious health effects, is becoming more widespread. Moreover, as in other parts of the world, the population has been exposed to other types of substance abuse agents, such as hashish and heroin. The abuse of prescription drugs such as amphetamines is a growing problem.

In the GCC population, the susceptibility to mind-altering drugs might resemble the susceptibility to substance abuse in persons living in other regions of the world. If so, then, as Al-Adawi points out, there is an urgent need to address the reasons for and the management of substance abuse in this region.

In chapter 6 Cother Hajat examines chronic disease and underlying risk factors in the GCC states, focusing on cardiovascular mortality, cancer mortality, diabetes, tobacco consumption, and obesity. Comparing these parameters with findings for the countries that are members of the Organization for Economic

Cooperation and Development is revealing. For example, obesity rates in the GCC states are among the world's highest, as are diabetes and cardiovascular disease. Smoking rates are lower and cancer rates are much lower, perhaps related to decreased smoking exposure.

Reducing the burden of diabetes and cardiovascular disease will require lowering obesity rates, either by modifying diet or increasing exercise. As we point out in our own contribution to the volume, chapter 7, on lifestyle diseases, this will require a massive effort involving individuals and multiple agencies within each country. It will also require a shift from thinking about disease treatment to disease prevention. Part of this change in thinking will be an individual responsibility, but equally important will be implementing changes in the healthcare system to initiate new and strengthen existing prevention programs by incorporating lifestyle medicine approaches, such as physical activity, stress reduction, smoking cessation, and healthy nutrition. Those with chronic diseases that cause debilitating pain and suffering can also benefit from evidence-based integrative (complementary) medicine modalities, such as mind–body techniques, dietary modifications, acupuncture, and other patient-centered human healing methods.[3] Integrative medicine treats the whole person, not just the disease.

Some populations of the GCC states have income levels several times higher than other parts of the world. These high income levels may be related to the current epidemic of lifestyle diseases—such as obesity, diabetes, and heart disease—that are so prevalent in this region. Chapter 7 discusses these illnesses, their rapid increase during the past few decades, and the potential for their control through public health measures. We point out that the current population is relatively young, but in the coming decades, with advancing age, the frequency of lifestyle diseases—especially diabetes, heart disease, strokes, and cancer—will rapidly increase, threatening to overwhelm the existing healthcare system.

Although not considered a true lifestyle disease, motor vehicle injury rates are higher in the GCC states than in Europe or the United States. These injuries are now the main cause of premature mortality throughout the region. Control is possible through stronger laws and more aggressive enforcement of existing laws. The key to reducing injury rates is political rather than medical.

There is a real potential for altering the growth trajectory for lifestyle diseases with comprehensive health promotion programs involving individuals, schools, and the region's respective governments. In the absence of effective programs, one estimate has projected the financial burden of lifestyle diseases in the GCC as $68 billion in 2022.[4]

The seven chapters in this book each cover a different topic, but there are several common overlapping themes. A special problem in the region relates to the large proportion of guest workers or expatriates—amounting to about half the total population. In some countries, such as Qatar, noncitizens constitute almost 80 percent of the population. Healthcare statistics generally are drawn from the native population, and thus only partially reflect the overall levels of health in the population. Also, the small size of the native population restricts the pool of native healthcare workers, resulting in a sustained need for foreign healthcare workers to satisfy the needs of the region.

Another problem dealt with in several chapters concerns the relative youth of the population. In many of the world's wealthy countries, birthrates are low and older persons form a majority of the population. The GCC states still have relatively youthful populations, with the result that conditions such as cancer and Alzheimer's disease are uncommon. Preparing for the transition from a younger to an older population will be a challenge facing each of the GCC states.

A major concern for the GCC is its preparation for the management of healthcare when its currently abundant energy resources are depleted. Recognizing this, the region is now focusing on educating the local population to assume the tasks that are now carried out by expatriates. New hospitals, such as the modern Sidra Medical and Research Center in Qatar, are under construction, and the region now has numerous medical schools whose aim is to train productive healthcare professionals who will remain within the region after completing their training. Nevertheless, it will require a strenuous effort for the region to be able to sustain a healthcare system without the help of foreign manpower.

The situation of healthcare in the GCC states continues to evolve. The emergence of lifestyle diseases, mental health conditions, the aging population, healthcare costs, health coverage, and a shortage of healthcare workforce personnel pose considerable challenges. Factors that are likely to shape and drive healthcare delivery in the years ahead include information and medical technology, regional and global partnerships, self-care, patient safety efforts, growing health awareness, government and hospital regulations, changing societal values and needs, and the changing face of the expatriate population. An interest in women's health, the adoption of new health technology, and the changing face of healthcare professionals' education are also receiving attention and are likely to influence the healthcare landscape in the GCC states.

The GCC's rapid economic growth has dramatically changed its healthcare systems and situation. Life expectancy, the human development index, and other health indicators have significantly improved. It took many decades for high-income European and North American nations, with their stable and growing economies, to enable their healthcare systems to mature. From this perspective, the GCC states have performed quite well in the health sector, in consideration of the comparatively very recent onset of economic development. The contents of this book remind us that a clear healthcare policy, with a focus on efficiency and equal access to resources, will be required to maintain and further improve the health and quality of life of the GCC's population.

NOTES

1. Economist Intelligence Unit, "The GCC in 2020: Resources for the Future," *The Economist*, 2010, http://graphics.eiu.com/upload/eb/GCC_in_2020_Resources_WEB.pdf.

2. See Mehran Kamrava, ed., *The Political Economy of the Persian Gulf* (New York: Oxford University Press, 2012).

3. Edzard Ernst, Max Pittler, Barbara Wider, and Kate Boddy, *Oxford Handbook of Complementary Medicine* (Oxford: Oxford University Press, 2008); David Reilly, "The Healing Shift Enquiry," www.davidreilly.net/HealingShift/Home.html.

4. Booz & Company, "The $68 Billion Challenge: Quantifying and Tackling the Burden of Chronic Diseases in the GCC," Strategy& (PricewaterhouseCoopers), December 5, 2013, www.strategyand.pwc.com/global/home/what-we-think/reports-white-papers/article-display/the-68-billion-dollar-challenge.

A HISTORICAL OVERVIEW OF HEALTHCARE IN THE GULF COOPERATION COUNCIL STATES

Nabil M. Kronfol

T his chapter outlines the historical transformation of the healthcare systems in the six countries of the Gulf Cooperation Council (GCC). This analysis is based on published articles and annual government reports. In addition, personal reminiscences from people who have been instrumental in developing regional healthcare services are included. It should be noted that the history of regional healthcare development, as important as it is, lacks documentation and published literature. It is hoped that this chapter will encourage officials who are in a position to participate in the documentation and analysis of these historic events.

The chapter describes four phases. The first phase narrates the beginning of health services at the turn of the twentieth century in all six GCC countries. The second phase describes the beginning of the development of the region's healthcare systems, which went on to become world-class modern systems by the end of the twentieth century. The third phase develops the current situation. The fourth and final phase is a discussion of the main determinants of the transformation of the healthcare systems and the current challenges faced by the GCC countries. This last phase draws from the perspectives of the chapter's author, who has lived through this period and who was often an actor in the transformation of these systems.

HISTORICAL OVERVIEW

Considering the health problems during the 1950s and 1960s, we generally assumed that every patient had five diseases before he came to the hospital complaining of yet another problem. The five diseases were malaria, trachoma, intestinal parasites, malnutrition, and anaemia. But what brought the patient to the hospital was usually something else, such as a broken bone, a serious burn, pneumonia, meningitis, tetanus, strangulated hernias, obstructed labour, intestinal obstruction, serious trauma such as camel bites or fishing accidents. . . . We rarely saw cases of appendicitis, gallbladder disease, gastric ulcers or heart attacks. Obesity was virtually unheard of. If we encountered these diseases, it was in a patient who had been off-loaded from a ship in the harbour or an individual who was not an Omani. But as prosperity came to the country and eating habits changed, all these diseases became common.[1]

The statement above was written by Dr. Donald Bosch, one of the first physicians to staff the American Mission Hospital in Oman, to describe many of the conditions that prevailed in the GCC countries at the end of the nineteenth century.

Bahrain

Health services in the Kingdom of Bahrain were established in the early twentieth century, with the American Mission Hospital in 1903. With a twenty-one-bed capacity (box 1.1), the hospital treated Bahrainis, and served other patients as well, many of whom traveled from the surrounding countries to seek medical treatment. Subsequently, the smaller memorial Victoria Hospital was established with a twelve-bed capacity and was "staffed by a general practitioner appointed by the British Government in India."[2] In 1925, the first government-run clinic was established, and was "staffed by an Indian doctor appointed by the government to treat injured pearl divers."[3] Subsequently, the Public Health Directorate, a preventive care agency, was established.

In 1936, a small hospital was established for the Bahrain Government Police Force, which was subsequently converted into isolation wards. With the discovery of oil in Bahrain in 1932, the Bahrain Petroleum Company established the first planned medical provision and constructed the thirty-seven-bed private Awali Hospital, especially for its staff; and then, in 1942, the first official government hospital, Al Naim Hospital, became operational.[4]

Box 1.1   **The Arabian Mission in Bahrain**

In 1888 at the Theological Seminary of the Dutch Reformed Church, in New Brunswick, New Jersey, a teacher and his three students had the calling to begin their work in Arabia. Dr. John G. Lansing had inherited his interest in Arabia from his father, a pioneer worker in Syria and Egypt. Born in Damascus, John Lansing had always felt the call back to Arabia. With the help of his three students—Samuel M. Zwemer, James Cantine, and Philip T. Phelps—he formulated a plan to create what was to become known as the Arabian Mission.

On May 23, 1888, the group signed their plan, arranged for their own funds. The Board of Foreign Missions passed their acceptance, and the Arabian Mission was born. Through the personal donations of several people, the Arabian Mission finally had enough money to send their first missionary out.

Samuel Zwemer stopped over in Bahrain and rented a room, which led to the opening of a medical dispensary in the Old Souk in 1883. This is how one man, Samuel Zwemer, ignited the vision of a health service for Bahrain with a single step. On January 26, 1903, after much hardship, the Mason Memorial Hospital in Bahrain was dedicated.

One hundred and eleven years later, the tradition of the missionaries and their service to the island of Bahrain still embodies the principles on which they serve the people of Bahrain.

Source: American Mission Hospital, www.amh.org.bh/history/.

Kuwait

Kuwait's first healthcare facilities date back to the early twentieth century. At the invitation of Sheikh Mubarak Al Sabah the Great, medical practitioners from the Arabian Mission of the Dutch Reformed Church in the United States established a hospital for men in 1911, and another for women in 1919.[5] In 1934, Olcott Memorial Hospital opened with thirty-four beds; and in 1936, the Ministry of Health (MOH) was established. Along with increased revenues from the oil industry, the government expanded the healthcare system, and in 1949 it opened the Amiri Hospital, and the Kuwait Oil Company established its own, smaller, facilities, so that "by 1950 general mortality had fallen to between seventeen and twenty-three per 1,000 population and infant mortality to between eighty and 100 per 1,000 live births."[6]

Oman

In the nineteenth century, the British operated early medical facilities in Muscat, mainly in relation to port quarantine services for Muscat Harbor.[7] The Muscat

Charitable Hospital, the first hospital in Oman, was constructed by the British Consulate in 1910, and was operational until 1970.[8] In the early twentieth century, the British government—along with a branch of the Reformed Church of America, the Arabian Mission—invested in larger healthcare facilities in Oman, establishing the Mutrah medicial clinic in 1904. In 1913, the American Mission opened a women's hospital in Muscat, and in 1934, a large general hospital called the American Mission Hospital. This was the only hospital in the country that was equipped with a functioning surgery unit, including an X-ray machine installed in 1940, with the capability to perform ten to twelve daily operations by 1950. Periodically, the American Mission was capable of sending physicians to travel around the country to visit, treat, and operate on patients in the interior regions. Over the course of its operations, several notable physicians—including Dr. Paul Harrison (1925–39), Dr. Wells Thorns (1939–70), and Dr. Donald Bosch (1955–74)—worked in Oman's growing healthcare field.[9]

Qatar

In Qatar, healthcare was mostly administered using traditional medicines and methods before the discovery of oil, where "barbers performed circumcisions and other minor procedures, and herbalists dispensed natural remedies."[10] In 1945, a small hospital was established, where only one physician oversaw operations; and later, in 1959, Rumailah Hospital, the first state hospital, was established, with 170 beds. A 165-bed maternity hospital opened in 1965.[11]

Saudi Arabia

Similar to the other Gulf states, Saudi Arabia's oil revenues enabled it to develop a modern healthcare system. Before the discovery of oil, healthcare mainly revolved around traditional medicines and practices.[12] In about the early twentieth century, in 1926, both the Ajyad Hospital in Mecca and the Bab Shareef Hospital in Jeddah were established, and the newly formed MOH oversaw eleven hospitals and medical dispensaries all around the country, as well as the first nursing school. In the same year, even though the country was still in its very early stages of development,[13] King Abdulaziz Al-Saud (1880–1953), formally decreed that the Saudi Arabian government was establishing a Health Department, which was named the General Directorate for Health and Aid and was under the supervision of the Bureau of the Attorney General.[14] Even though traditional healthcare was still practiced by much of the population, this directorate oversaw the construction of a series of medical facilities in many urbanizing areas that aided in controlling disease and raising the standards of the kingdom's available health services.[15]

In 1925, a royal decree by King Abdulaziz led to the establishment of the first public health department in Mecca,[16] and in 1949 more medical facilities were opened, creating and attracting a larger number of healthcare professionals.[17] In 1950, the MOH was able to transform and develop Saudi Arabia's health sector, despite the fact that the economy remained underdeveloped and funds were low.[18]

In the 1950s, organized preventive health services in Saudi Arabia began in earnest. In al-Qatif and al-Hassa Oasis in the Eastern Province, the MOH, the Saudi Arabian Oil Company (Aramco), and the World Health Organization (WHO) launched the first campaign against malaria, which was a success. This led to the adoption of the malaria control program in other provinces. It was not until the 1960s that healthcare development began rapid improvements; and by the 1980s, there was a well-developed and modern healthcare system. Subsequently, the government created five-year development plans to oversee the growth of the sector, which became significantly improved.[19] Serious improvements in healthcare have been achieved in Saudi Arabia since then.

The United Arab Emirates

The United Arab Emirates remained underdeveloped in the years leading up to the discovery of oil. The poor relied on traditional medicines and practices for their healthcare needs, and wealthy patients could opt to travel to neighboring countries for treatment. Britain became interested in the United Arab Emirates' welfare as a result of the successes achieved by the US missionaries in Muscat and Bahrain, and it appointed a medical officer for the Trucial Coast in 1938, followed by an Indian physician serving in a dispensary in Dubai.

In 1943, in the Al Ras area of Dubai, the local community received modest healthcare services from a general medical practitioner based in a small healthcare center, and by 1949 the British government had established Al Maktum Hospital, which was overseen by a British physician from the Indian Medical Service. The Kuwait, Iran, and the Trucial States Development Fund contributed to the country's healthcare development, increasing the number of beds to 157 during 1973. The American Mission established hospitals in Sharjah, Al Ain, and Ras al Khaymahin in the 1950s and 1960s. During the 1970s, with the federation of the United Arab Emirates, medical services were advanced, along

---

Box 1.2 **The Oasis Hospital in Al Ain**

What changed the course of the history of medicine in the United Arab Emirates was the impetus from the two sheikhs to provide adequate healthcare for their community. They had been impressed by facilities at American-run hospitals they had visited in Bahrain and Muscat in the 1950s and were keen to match their standards on home turf.

On November 20, 1960, the American Dr. Mariam Kennedy arrived with her husband, Pat, also a doctor, and their young children, Kathleen, Nancy, Scott, and Douglas. They were later joined by other Christian missionaries from the United States and Canada. The Kennedys set up base in a mud-block guest house donated by Sheikh Zayed and had not even unpacked when their first maternity patient arrived two days later. Aptly, the baby was called Mubarak, meaning the blessed, and word soon spread among the neighboring villages. Patients would travel for days by camel, donkey, and on foot to see Mariam and Pat Kennedy, camping on the grounds until they could be seen and offering to pay with animals and eggs when they lacked financial means. Often the sheikhs would foot the medical bill, a legacy that continues to this day. Theirs is the only hospital we know of that does not refuse patients, says Printy. Within two months, there were more than two hundred patients arriving every morning.

Source: Tahira Yaqoob, "How Missionaries Transformed Abu Dhabi Health Care," *The National*, November 5, 2010, www.thenational.ae/news/uae-news/health/how-missionaries -transformed-abu-dhabi -healthcare#full.

---

with several hospitals in the larger urban centers of Abu Dhabi, Dubai, Ras al Khaimah, Sharjah, and Dibba, as well as smaller clinics in the towns, rural areas, and villages. A private facility in Abu Dhabi, the Oasis, was the first to receive the Joint Commission International Accreditation in 2007 (box 1.2).

HEALTH SERVICES BEFORE THE TWENTY-FIRST CENTURY

The twenty-first century has witnessed the development of government-run health services in all the GCC states—a move from the initial missionary and benevolent medical services to a comprehensive health system based on primary healthcare with fully operational inpatient facilities. This development of the health sector has been in parallel to state building since independence, and has moved toward modern patterns of service that have prevailed since the end of World War II.

Bahrain

Again, with the discovery of oil in the early 1930s, Bahrain's economy was transformed, with abundant wealth and prosperity brought to the nation. At the time when the first census was carried out in Bahrain in 1941, the country's total population was 89,970, including 74,040 Bahrainis and 15,930 expatriate residents. By 1959, the population had grown to 143,135, an increase of 59.1 percent in less than twenty years. This growth can be attributed largely to the improvement in health services in Bahrain, which alleviated the spread of contagious diseases and improved the population's general health. Bahrain joined the WHO in May 1967, and since then it has played a major role in implementing the resolutions of this international organization. Comprehensive health services are provided to the whole country, according to the WHO's global objectives in which most of the healthcare services are provided by the MOH. Primary healthcare (PHC) is the most significant sector of the public health services. PHC is provided to all citizens in Bahrain at twenty PHC centers and three clinics that have been developed in line with the Declaration of Alma Ata in 1978.[20]

With Bahrain's massive increases in population and expanding economy, it was necessary to develop a large modern hospital to meet the country's healthcare needs, and thus the Salmaniya Hospital was constructed in 1957, renovated in 1978, expanded into a teaching hospital for the Arabian Gulf University in 1984, and developed into the Salmaniya Medical Complex in 1997. In-patient care is also provided by the psychiatric hospital, with 201 beds; by the geriatric hospital, with 101 beds; and by four maternity hospitals, with 241 beds. The Ministry of Defense established the Bahrain Defence Force Hospital, with 349 beds, which provides specialized services to members of the Bahrain Defence Force and their families. The Shaikh Mohammed Al-Khalifa Cardiac Centre further provides advanced cardiac care to Bahrain's people.[21]

Bahrain has eight private hospitals, with a number of others at various stages of development, including the Bahrain International Hospital, with 100 beds; the American Mission Hospital, with 40 beds; and the Awali Hospital of the Bahrain National Oil Company, with 37 beds. The College of Health Sciences, inaugurated in 1976, is operated by qualified and skilled faculty members, and is considered the only institution in Bahrain capable of providing educational programs for nursing and allied health professionals. Allied health education is offered at the associate degree level, and nursing education is offered at the associate and bachelor's degree levels. The Arabian Gulf University was established by the six Gulf countries in 1979, and comprises the Medicine and Medical Sciences, Applied Sciences, and Education colleges. The College of Medicine and Medical Sciences has adopted a modern and innovative approach to medical education, and other postbasic specializations include the Specialty Training Residency Program in Medical Specializations for Doctors in 1999, which prepares Bahraini doctors for the Arab Board Certification examination in a variety of medical and surgical specialties. Other private higher educational institutions include the Medical University of Bahrain, which is operated and managed by the Royal College of Surgeons in Ireland, and Ahlia University, which offers a BS program in physiotherapy.[22]

Relaying his most significant achievements as minister of health and minister of education in Bahrain, Dr. Ali Fakhro noted:

> I was in the Health Ministry from 1970 to 1982 and in that time we made some significant changes. When I first started, the ministry consisted of mostly foreign staff including doctors and nurses. When I left the ministry it was fully staffed with Bahrainis. We established the College of Health Sciences, the first of its kind in the Arab world, to train nurses and health technicians. This was a key step in accelerating the Bahrainization of ministry staff. We prioritized public health services and preventive programs resulting in the elimination of malaria, typhoid and dysentery as well as the reduction of infectious childhood diseases by more than two-thirds. We prioritized primary healthcare by establishing health centers within three kilometers of every citizen's home. We established the College of Medicine as part of the Arabian Gulf University. We initiated the Education and Training Program for family doctors, the first of its kind in the Arab world. We proposed the establishment of the Arab Board of Health Specializations to the Health Ministers' Council for GCC states and proceeded to win the approval of Arab health ministers. I was eventually appointed chair of the board and its executive committee for 15 years. As minister of education from 1982 to 1995, I also made significant achievements. We established the first national university in Bahrain. We contributed to the establishment of the Arabian Gulf University, which is the regional university for GCC states. The two ministries were managed by a committee and chaired by the minister. They included senior officials, specialists and consultants, and this resulted in a democratic, consultative and cooperative system.[23]

Kuwait

In the 1950s a comprehensive healthcare system was introduced to the country by the Kuwaiti government, which was capable of offering free services to the population; in fact, healthcare benefited from ranking third in the national budget, after public works and education. The healthcare sector, like many others in the country, needed and attracted a large international workforce, with most of the physicians being foreigners. With these new, systematized services, there were dramatic improvements in public health, including infant and child mortality rates, as well as the population's overall life expectancy.[24]

Seventy-two health centers and specialized clinics administer PHC, secondary healthcare is offered through six general hospitals, and tertiary healthcare is provided through a variety of national specialized hospitals and clinics. The efficient delivery of health services has improved through the regionalization of the health system in six health regions; and in 1999, health insurance for expatriates was legislated.

Oman

In 1958, small government medical services began in Oman, largely in response to a development subsidy from the British government, with several dispensaries and health centers in the interior, a small military hospital in the capital, and a mobile clinic with touring medical service. Up until the 1970s, healthcare services were small and basic, and were largely dominated by services offered by the American Mission Hospital. This was the country's only general hospital, and one that was struggling under its patient load and conditions of underdevelopment. Electricity shortages and lack of air-conditioning meant that any elective surgery was postponed from the summer months to the winter.[25] These issues were mildly alleviated when the hospital installed a generator in 1964, allowing for the number of operations to increase by 23 percent, to 2,385; and for the number of eye operations to increase by 50 percent, to 985.[26] From 1968 to 1969, more patients began to be treated, and the load of outpatient cases increased by 30 percent, to 51,800.

In the years before 1958, it was customary for people to travel for several days to reach one of the already-crowded hospitals, which were serviced by a total of thirteen physicians—a physician–population ratio of 1 to 50,000.[27] In 1970, the average life expectancy was only 49.3 years, and morbidity and mortality rates were high, with one out of every eight infants born dying within their first year, and one out of every five dying before reaching their fifth birthday. Malaria was prevalent, with one of every three people experiencing an episode; and out of every thousand, thirty were infected with trachoma, eight with pulmonary tuberculosis, and six with hepatitis.

In 1970s, Oman's modernization and development began in earnest, but it was only with the accession of Sultan Qaboos in the 1980s that a systematized, basic healthcare infrastructure was made available to the population, with significant effects on the country's health development. In just three decades, the infant mortality rate has dropped to only one-fifth of its value, and the under-five mortality rate to one-sixth. Currently, these rates are just 16.2 and 19.7 per 1,000 live births, down from 118 and 181, respectively, and the average life span in Oman has also dramatically increased, from forty-nine years in 1970 to seventy-four years today. Oman's health indicators have approached the levels found in the countries that belong to the Organization for Economic Cooperation and Development.[28] The implementation of health policies and strategies has resulted in rapid and significant changes in health and mortality patterns. In 2000, the WHO ranked Oman 1st among all its 191 member states in health attainment levels, and 8th in health system performance.

Similar to the other GCC countries, Oman's main health problems are shifting from communicable diseases to health problems related to changes in lifestyle. The Omani MOH's policy is to encourage investment by the private sector in the health sector, but the government's provision of services has limited the private sector's development, and hence also that of health insurance. Because the government-funded system provides low-cost healthcare services, the private system faces very stiff competition. In 2001, assessing the outcomes of government investments in the public sector, an independent nationwide survey found that 70 percent of the public was satisfied with the health system.

In 1959, at the American Missionary Hospital, a missionary nurse began training nationals locally in nursing practices. In 1970, a missionary school for nursing—Arrahma Nursing School, within Arrahma Hospital—was established as Oman's first health-training institute, and it allowed students with a minimal primary education to enroll. In 1972, five nurses graduated, and eighty-three graduated between 1972 and 1981, when the MOH began overseeing the school. Soon thereafter, other types of training were also offered, including courses for medical laboratory technicians. Medical education became increasingly systematized—Oman's Medical College was accredited by the University of West Virginia in the United States; and the MD degree was offered by the

Sultan Qaboos University, with accreditation by the United Kingdom's General Medical Counsel.

Qatar

Qatar established its first general hospital, Rumaillah Hospital, in the late 1950s, with a capacity of two hundred beds. In 1972, with the accession of Sheikh Khalifa bin Hamad, there was rapid development in the healthcare sector, and the Hamad Medical Corporation (HMC) was established in 1979, with high-technology, modern facilities; a network of PHC centers; and four specialized hospitals. These investments, however, were subject to the drop in oil prices, and 10 percent of the HMC's staff was cut in 1986.

The MOH and HMC organize the country's healthcare system, with the MOH being responsible for administrative, regulatory, and policy matters. In 1969, the School of Nursing was established, and it enrolled students from the intermediate school level but was not able to meet the demand for nurses.[29] In later years, Weill Cornell Medicine was invited to open a medical college and research facilities at Qatar's "Education City," and nursing education was provided by Qatar University (at the BSc level) and the Ministry of Public Health, which graduates diploma-level nurses through the Secondary Technical School of Nursing.[30] Despite these efforts, only 8.4 percent of Qatari nurses make up the total nurse force.[31]

Saudi Arabia

In the 1950s, Aramco collaborated with the WHO and the MOH to battle malaria in the eastern part of the kingdom, as well as a variety of other campaigns to control bilharziasis, leishmaniasis, trachoma, tuberculosis, and other endemic diseases in other parts of the country.[32] From 1970 to 1980, most of the healthcare services were largely curative, and were administered through a network of hospitals and dispensaries, and episodic outbreaks of diseases were controlled through health offices.

Saudi adopted PHC in 1978 as the basis of its health delivery system, followed by the integration of health centers, dispensaries, and maternal and child health centers in 1980. In addition to the efforts of the MOH, other government units—including the Ministry of Defense, the National Guard, and the Interior Ministry—further provided comprehensive curative healthcare services

in many of the major urban areas. In order to encourage the growth and pro-
fessionalization of the local healthcare sector, the government gave hundreds
of scholarships to high school graduates to study medicine and allied health
sciences abroad.[33] Moreover, in 1967 King Saud University was established in
Riyadh, and it was affiliated with the London College of Medicine; medical
colleges were opened within King Abdul-Aziz University and King Faisal University in 1975; King Saud University opened a branch college in Abha in 1980,
which was transformed into King Khalid University; and Umm Al-Qura University was established in 1996. Despite these efforts, few Saudi nationals were
working in the medical field, making up less than 20 percent of the physicians
working in the country.[34]

In addition to government services, the rapidly growing private sector provides basic medical care as well as highly organized specialist services in a number of private hospitals, clinics, dispensaries, and pharmacies, which are mostly
located in the larger cities.

In addition to the everyday Saudi healthcare needs, during the hajj season,
preventive and curative healthcare services are provided for all pilgrims. The
MOH organizes various measures during the hajj, which attracts a large number
(1.3 million) of pilgrims, a large proportion of whom are elderly, who bring
their own public health challenges.[35]

The United Arab Emirates

Even though the United Arab Emirates is made up of seven emirates, its most
advanced healthcare services are concentrated in Dubai and Abu Dhabi, under
the supervision of, respectively, the Dubai Health Authority and the Abu Dhabi
Health Authority. The Northern emirates—Sharjah, Ajman, Ras al Khaimah,
and Fujairah—do not have as many facilities as Dubai and Abu Dhabi. In 1951,
Al Maktoum Hospital was inaugurated, followed by Rashid Hospital (454 beds)
in 1973, Dubai Hospital (625 beds) in 1983, and Al Wasl Hospital (367 beds,
in the Maternity and Pediatric Specialized Hospital) in 1986. In addition to
these larger hospitals, a variety of clinics and health centers are located all over
the emirates. In 1970, the Department of Health and Medical Services became
operational, and it oversaw the modernization and development of healthcare
in Dubai.[36]

In the early years of Abu Dhabi's healthcare development, it received technical and material assistance from Egypt. In 1965, only one physician was
employed by the Abu Dhabi government, and three others were employed in

private practice. In 1971, after federation, the health system was characterized by rapid growth but a simultaneous lack of coordination among the different institutions, and also among the different emirates. In the 1990s, great improvements were made in the public healthcare system, and the various oil companies and the military operated their own private medical facilities. Although Abu Dhabi and Dubai have most of the advanced facilities, the other emirates are provided with government-run facilities and hospitals. Increasingly, the private sector has been developed, and has formed partnerships with state-run services to provide the people of the United Arab Emirates with comprehensive healthcare. The private sector contributes to preventive and curative services through a network of hospitals, clinics, and medical centers.[37]

THE CURRENT SITUATION

The healthcare sectors of the GCC states have come a long way, and the governments of these countries now run modern, state-of-the-art facilities and systems that concentrate on the principal causes of morbidity and mortality. The populations of the GCC are now less afflicted by communicable diseases, and instead are affected by the diseases of prosperity—such as diabetes and obesity, traffic accidents, and ailments associated with old age and occupational health. Over the years, there has been an increase in initiatives encouraging partnerships with the private sector, and the provision of healthcare has increasingly moved away from paternalistic perceptions to become a human right, acknowledged through government legislation.

Oman

Oman's modern healthcare systems were established in the 1970s, along with the reign of Sultan Qaboos. During the past four decades, health has become a primary concern as a result of Oman's prosperity and social and economic progress.[38] In 2000, the WHO ranked Oman's health system 1st for its overall performance, and 8th for its health system performance, among 191 member countries.[39]

As a result of the effective implementation of national health programs, between 1991 and 2005 there was a rapidly declining trend in the epidemiological situation of communicable diseases in Oman. In the past, before 1970, communicable diseases—including diarrheal diseases, cholera, malaria, tuberculosis, and trachoma—were the most common ailments. In the 1970s and 1980s, one of the most prevalent public health concerns was malaria. In 1999, according to the MOH, Oman experienced its last "indigenous" case of malaria.[40] In 2004, 615 cases of malaria were reported in Oman, and another 544 were reported in 2005; but these were all imported from East Africa and the Indian subcontinent.[41]

Oman's implementation of a series of healthcare reforms has meant that the overall health of the Omani people has improved dramatically.[42] During the past four decades, greater economic prosperity has transformed the epidemiological patterns of diseases in Oman, with chronic diseases now being the most dominant (see table 1.1).[43]

Oman's MOH has faced a series of challenges in order to modernize the national healthcare system since the 1970s,[44] and in response it has organized five-year health development plans, the first of which was instituted in 1976.[45] The country's health policy has been committed to the global Health for All strategy, which it has implemented through a total of seven five-year plans. In the 1990s, a planning agency was set up, and health services were decentralized through allocation to ten health regions, in which local health administrations were set up at the *wilayat* (province) level. This was a period of growth in the healthcare sector in which several hospitals, health centers, and preventive programs were established.[46]

Since the 1970s, education has contributed significantly to the country's growth. In 1986, Sultan Qaboos University was established; and in 1993, the first physicians graduated from the university's College of Medicine. Subsequently, the Oman Medical College, a new private medical school, was established in partnership with West Virginia University's School of Medicine. In addition, continuing medical education programs were established in all hospitals, as well as other specialty groupings that regularly organize a series of conferences and workshops. In 1994, the Oman Medical Specialty Board was established as a supervisory institution overseeing all postgraduate medical training programs in Oman, including new residency training programs, and nursing and allied health science institutes.[47]

Similar to the situation in the other GCC states, Oman's workforce was dominated by foreigners only four decades ago; but due to government policies in relation to healthcare education and practice, the representation of Omanis in the MOH workforce was significant, with a rapid increase in the number of local physicians, nurses, and laboratory technicians.[48] The government sector, including university practice, employs approximately 80 percent of all physicians and 90 percent of all specialists. The MOH is the main accreditation body

Table 1.1 **Epidemiological Trend for Selected Diseases in Oman, 1991–2005**

Disease	1991	2005
Malaria	19,274	544
Tuberculosis	405	257
Measles	220	19
Hypertension	2,502	2,167
Diabetes	2,072	4,117
Heart disease	4,077	5,640
Cancer	2,215	3,382

Source: Data from S. S. Ganguly, M. A. Al-Shafaee, J. A. Al-Lawati, P. K. Dutta, and K. K. Duttagupta, "Epidemiological Transition of Some Diseases in Oman: A Situational Analysis," *Eastern Mediterranean Health Journal* 15, no. 1 (January–February 2009).

regulating the private practice sector, and it has permitted senior specialists to engage in private practice after their regular office hours.

Even though the nursing profession remained unattractive to Omani nationals up until the early 1980s, the MOH was able to attract more people into the profession by establishing a nursing college in every Omani *wilaya*, and by using the regional health facilities for training. This was especially beneficial for Omani girls, who no longer needed to travel for training but were able to study nursing near their homes. Further introductions of undergraduate and graduate programs in nursing has meant that this pattern is being accelerated and reinforced in all the GCC states. Although medical schools were initially established by the government in all the GCC states, during the past two decades there has been an increase in medical colleges established by the private sector as well as in nationals traveling abroad for their medical education. Upon their return, these physicians have assumed leadership positions in both private medical institutions and councils, as well as in the government healthcare system.

Today, the MOH is Oman's main healthcare provider and regulator, providing free healthcare for all Omanis and expatriate government employees and their dependents.[49] In 1987, the flagship of the MOH's network, the Royal Hospital, was established, with 630 beds. The first general hospital to be built by the MOH was the Khoula Hospital, with 428 beds, which is now a referral center for neurosurgery, plastic and reconstructive surgery, and trauma and orthopedics. Al Nahdah Hospital, with 95 beds, was established as a specialist center for eye and otolaryngological disorders. In 1990, Sultan Qaboos University Hospital was opened, with a capacity of 532 beds.[50]

Other than the MOH, government entities such as the defense and security forces provide free healthcare services for employees and their dependents, while expatriates employed in private institutions depend on the private health sector and are normally covered by private health insurance or directly through their companies, which in many cases are responsible for the provision of healthcare.

In the early 1970s, after the accession of Sultan Qaboos, well-educated and professional Omani citizens were encouraged to return from their studies or domicile abroad to assume leadership roles in the healthcare system, leading to a largely stable local sector under the supervision of experienced nationals steering the government agencies and ministries. Many of these Omani professionals had been working or studying in the United Kingdom or in East Africa and could not return to Oman before the accession of Sultan Qaboos.

Qatar

Qatar has seen tremendous progress in its healthcare sector, which has become a leading example of state-of-the-art service provision and facilities. The scope of health services coverage has expanded, along with a number of primary health centers and hospitals throughout the country. In 2005, the National Health Authority was established to provide medical preventive and treatment services and to oversee public health services both locally and for Qatari nationals seeking medical treatment abroad. It also regulates the marketing and manufacturing of drugs in accordance with international quality standards. The organization also oversees Hamad Medical Corporation, Hamad Specialist and Educational Hospital, laboratories, private medical facilities, pharmacies, and PHC centers, and the like. The National Health Authority—and its successor, the Supreme Council of Health (SCH)—coordinate with the Health Insurance System to enhance health services and dissemination of health education and awareness, and undertake the organization of the private medical sector. The SCH is the highest regulatory healthcare authority in Qatar, and also oversees medical facilities in the private sector.[51]

Qatar's Hamad Medical Corporation, which was established in 1982, has become one of the region's most distinguished specialized medical institutions, supervising Hamad General Hospital (616 beds), Rumailah Hospital (362 beds), Women's Hospital (334 beds), Al-Khor Hospital, Al-Amal Oncology Hospital, Heart Hospital (120 beds), Al Wakrah Hospital (350 beds), and the Cuban Hospital in Dukhan.[52] The private health sector—including 219 private complexes and clinics, and four multispecialty hospitals—has become increasingly central to the country's overall healthcare system. The Al-Ahli Specialized Hospital, for example, is a 250-bed private hospital that has become central to the population's healthcare needs.[53]

The Qatari government's goal of improving the health of the country's population has been etched into its National Vision 2030, with an outline of establishing a high-quality healthcare system. In 2013, Law No. 7 was issued, enacting the National Health Insurance Scheme, which is a national health insurance program accessible to all citizens, residents, and visitors. The Health Insurance Law tasks the SCH with the responsibility for, and the supervision and development of, the National Health Insurance Scheme and the National Health Insurance Company, as well as with the "actual implementation and management" of the National Health Insurance Scheme.[54] The National Health Insurance Company is a government institution with a board of directors consisting of representatives from the SCH, the Ministry of Finance, the Ministry of Labour, the Ministry of the Interior, and the Central Municipality Council, as well as two members from the private business sector.

Saudi Arabia

The Saudi Arabian government has invested heavily in the kingdom's healthcare services, leading to a dramatic improvement in the quantity and quality of health and health services during the past few decades.[55] As Gallagher has stated, "although many nations have seen sizable growth in their healthcare systems, probably no other nation (other than Saudi Arabia) of large geographic expanse and population has, in comparable time, achieved so much on a broad national scale, with a relatively high level of care made available to virtually all segments of the population."[56]

Saudi Arabia has made serious improvements in the organization of its healthcare system, which have brought health services to people all over country.[57] About 60 percent of health services are delivered by the MOH, 20 percent is provided through other government agencies, and the remaining 20 percent is administered by the rapidly growing nongovernmental sector.[58] Increasingly, well-known Western companies are entering into joint ventures with national healthcare management organizations. The main health issues currently affecting Saudi Arabia include communicable diseases such as malaria and schistosomiasis, ailments related to the various psychological and environmental stresses of modern life, and injuries resulting from motor vehicle accidents.[59]

Even though the WHO reports that the Saudi healthcare system is ranked 26th among the world's 190 health systems, it still faces a number of challenges, including the lack of local Saudi healthcare professionals, such as physicians, nurses, and pharmacists. Because the majority of health personnel are expatriates, this leads to instability in the workforce, with a high rate of turnover. The healthcare system is also challenged by the MOH's many different roles and its budgetary concerns, along with the changing patterns of disease, the demand for free services, limited access to some to healthcare facilities, and a lack of national health awareness.[60]

The Saudi health system's ultimate aim is to provide comprehensive and integrated healthcare for the population; but to reduce the wasting of human and financial resources, there needs to be more effective coordination among stakeholders.[61] The Council of Health Services, which was established in 2002 and is headed by the minister of health, seeks to better integrate and develop Saudi healthcare service authorities.[62] It includes representatives from both the government and private health sectors.[63] In 1999, the Council for Cooperative Health Insurance was established by the government to respond to growing healthcare demand and to supervise a health insurance strategy.[64] In cooperation with other healthcare providers, and supervised by the Council of Health Services, the MOH is overseeing a twenty-year plan for implementing the national strategy for healthcare services.[65] Further, private health insurance is available through insurance firms covering different services. A parastatal body called the Insurance Corporation is accountable to the minister of health and is responsible for regulating the private sector.

Saudi Arabia's medical education sector has been significantly developed, with an increase in the number of medical colleges from five to twenty-one, with a variety of innovative as well as more traditional medical curricula and community-oriented programs. Both the private sector and the government have been supporting and investing in higher-education medical institutions and colleges. With the aim of introducing greater quality assurance, the National Commission for Academic Assessment and Accreditation was established in 2005 as an accreditation body for higher education institutes.[66]

Since 1975 both local and international businesses have been encouraged by various incentives to invest in the country's health sector. Policymakers and researchers regard privatization of public hospitals as a means of reforming the Saudi healthcare system.[67] Past failures in public-sector healthcare have spurred the Saudi government to invite private investors and private equity firms to help professionalize the field.[68] Despite these many investments in the construction of medical institutions, however, Saudi Arabia's healthcare sector still suffers from a shortage of human resources.[69]

All health-related activities are monitored by and fall under the control of the MOH, which is coming under increased pressure given its many institutional demands.[70] To relieve some of the burden, regional directorates have been given more autonomy to engage in their own administrative activities—whether planning, recruiting staff, formulating agreements, or making financial decisions.

In recent decades, to improve the management of some hospitals, the MOH has standardized an autonomous hospital system for thirty-one public hospitals across the country.[71] In addition, the MOH has engaged in a variety of different strategies to improve the management of these public institutions. Some of these strategies include direct operation by the MOH; partial operation by healthcare companies; cooperation with international governments, such the Netherlands, Germany, and Thailand; comprehensive operation by healthcare companies; and the autonomous hospital system.[72]

In 1982, Aramco was among the first to initiate quality assurance programs in Saudi Arabia, which was innovative for the time,[73] and was further emulated by King Faisal Specialist Hospital.[74] Since it began operations in 1975, the King Faisal Specialist Hospital and Research Center Services was managed by the Hospital Corporation of America. In 1985, management of the hospital was transferred to the Saudi authorities; and in 2000, it was accredited for its Quality Assurance Program by the Joint Commission on Accreditation of Hospitals.[75] In addition, in the 1990s, the MOH began implementing total quality management in hospitals, in cooperation with the Hospital Administration Development, a US organization.[76] And then, in 2000, the MOH also created the General Directorate of Quality Assurance.[77] To aid in the accreditation process for both public and private health services, the Central Board of Accreditation for Healthcare Institutions was established by the MOH in 2006.[78]

The United Arab Emirates

Similar to the other GCC states, the United Arab Emirates' health services have been tremendously improved during the past few decades since the establishment of the federation.[79] Commitment to heath has been central to the country's Constitution, which assures comprehensive, high-quality healthcare as a right for all citizens and residents. In 1986, Cabinet Decree No. 39 emphasized the PHC principles of equity, accessibility, acceptability, and community participation, and set in motion a national health strategy and work plan by declaring that PHC was essential to achieving the goal of Health for All by 2000. This was a new strategy to reshape the healthcare system, using an integrated health services approach to strengthen intrasectoral and intersectoral collaboration and to provide the population of the United Arab Emirates with effective and high-quality healthcare (box 1.3).[80]

DISCUSSION

Before independence in the 1970s, most GCC countries were characterized by poor health indicators and by an acute scarcity of professional human resources in the healthcare sector. It was only after the 1970s that concerted efforts began to develop the region's health systems under the leadership of national governments. The implementation of these plans was only possible because of national social and economic development agendas, in which the nation's health was a priority. This contributed to increased health coverage, leading to improved health outcomes overall, which has been most clearly reflected in increased life expectancy and in a reduction of morbidity and mortality (table 1.2). In addition, by building on existing employer-based insurance programs and expanding their coverage, GCC governments have contributed to the development of a variety of social protection programs for various categories of workers.[81]

In many cases, the GCC governments adopted and adapted the health systems that had been put in place by the former colonial powers, which generally belonged to the public sector, and which were characterized by a "paternalistic" perspective on healthcare. GCC governments offered healthcare services to their constituencies in what could be considered a charitable donation rather than as a citizen's right. These curative facilities were developed by the GCC governments as measures to protect their societies—including such programs and facilities as quarantines; healthcare legislation; environmental sanitation services; and efforts to protect people from communicable and infectious diseases, such as tuberculosis, cholera, leprosy, and smallpox.

Since gaining independence, the GCC countries have used their oil revenues to invest in the complete reform, modernization, and development of the public-sector welfare system, beginning with the construction of inpatient facilities. In the early years, these were mostly operated by invited international hospital management companies, which was a means of providing high-quality medical services to a rapidly increasing population of nationals and expatriates in a short period. Subsequently, along with a gradual transfer of knowledge and a

Box 1.3   **Dubai Health Authority Timeline**

1943   Opening of a small healthcare center in the Al Ras area
1951   The first phase of the Al Maktoum Hospital is built
1952–73   The construction of the Al Maktoum Hospital is completed, with 157 beds
1972   Establishment of the Department of Health and Medical Services
1972   Rashid Hospital is opened in Dubai, complete with 454 beds
1975   Seven community clinics are opened in Dubai to reach out to the people
1978   The Central Services Complex is established
1983   Dubai Hospital opens, equipped with 625 beds
1986   Al Wasl Hospital, a 367-bed facility specializing in maternity and pediatric care, is
            inaugurated. In 2012 the name of Al Wasl Hospital is changed to Latifa Hospital
1988–95   Six community health centers are opened
1998   The concept of primary healthcare is established and adopted. Twenty health cen-
            ters are opened across Dubai to ensure access to basic primary healthcare
2007   The Dubai Health Authority is formed

Sources: Government of Dubai, www.dha.gov.ae/En/aboutus/pages/ourhistory.aspx; www.dha.gov.ae
/En/aboutus/Pages/AboutUs.aspx.

Table 1.2   **Change in Public Health Indicators in the GCC**

Indicator	Bahrain 1970	Bahrain 2005	Kuwait 1970	Kuwait 2005	Oman 1970	Oman 2005	Qatar 1970	Qatar 2005	Saudi Arabia 1970	Saudi Arabia 2005	United Arab Republic 1970	United Arab Republic 2005
LEB	69.5	74.8	74.9	77.5	69	74.3	72.2	75.8	71	73.6	70	72.6
IMR	20.0	7.6	12.1	8.2	25	10.3	19	8.1	170	18.6	12	8.1
<5 CMR	22	10.1	16	10	30	11.1	25	9	34	21.7	14	10.2
MMR	60	1	7.3	4	150	15.4	8.3	7	41	12	30	1
CBR	27.7	—	24.8	—	43.7	—	24.7	—	49	—	23.8	—
CDR	3.1	—	2.4	—	4.9	—	3.7	—	23	—	2.8	—
TFR	3.8	—	3.4	—	7.4	—	3.1	—	4.3	—	4.1	—
THE per capita	463	—	537	—	136	—	1397	—	—	—	767	—
THE as % of GDP	4.8	—	3.9	—	3	—	3	—	—	—	3.5	—
THE public %	8.8	—	78	—	80	—	75	—	6	—	77	—
MD/10,000	5.56	27.6	10	18	0.4	17.9	8.3	27.6	1.7	20	1.65	16.1
Nurses	23	—	4.4	—	26	—	3.5	—	1.0	—	3.6	—

Source: Data from Abdel Latif, "Aspiring to Build Health Services and Systems Led by Primary Health Care in the Eastern Mediterranean Region," *Eastern Mediterranean Health Journal* 14, special issue, 2008.

Note: LEB, life expectancy at birth in years; IMR, infant mortality rate per 1,000 live births (LBs); < 5 CMR under-5 mortality rate for children per 1,000 live births; MMR, maternal mortality rate per 100,000 live births; CBR, crude birthrate; CDR, crude death rate; THE, total health expenditures.

maturation of the medical market, each country's national health authority took over the management of these institutions.

In 1978, most of the region's countries adopted the Declaration of Alma Ata, which allowed them effectively to build their healthcare systems on the basis of PHC, along with its philosophy, concepts, programs, and referral system.[82] Currently, there are various networks of modern PHC centers all over the region. These are largely staffed by graduates of family medicine programs that were simultaneously introduced in the region, beginning with Lebanon and Bahrain with the family medicine programs at the American University of Beirut and the MOH in Bahrain, in cooperation with the American University of Beirut. Even before it adopted the Alma Ata Declaration, in 1976 Bahrain based its healthcare system on PHC.

In 1975, the Secretariat of the Gulf Ministers of Health was established at a meeting in Riyadh in order to enhance regional cooperation between the Gulf countries (box 1.4). The seven Gulf countries, including Iraq at the time, began engaging in regional cooperation programs. These include the shared purchasing of medicines and medical supplies, which meant significant discounts, and which as joint programs are still operational. The secretariat also supported a variety of education programs for the maintenance of medical equipment and to monitor quality standards for nursing and allied health professionals.

Securing self-sufficiency in human resources development became a priority for all the GCC states, and this became reflected in national commitments to invest in medical, pharmacy, and nursing schools we well as allied personnel throughout the region. In 1950, there was only one medical school in Saudi Arabia, but this had increased to thirty-five by the end of 2005 (see table 1.3). In 1970, there was an acute shortage of human resources across the region, but by 2005 most countries welcomed an increase in physicians, dentists, and pharmacists (see table 1.4).

The private sector has been increasingly involved in the provision of medical education and medical care since the mid-1980s. The GCC governments issued a variety of incentives to private investors, including tax cuts, to operate a variety of direct and indirect ventures, which saw a rapid growth in the private sector's role in service delivery of health education, and major health-sector reforms in many countries of the region. The private sector played a greater role and maximized flexibility, managerial capacities, and entrepreneurship. In the twenty-first century, many countries joined the World Trade Organization in an effort to promote privatization and to encourage the growth of medical

---

Box 1.4   **The Health Ministers' Council for the GCC**

The Health Ministers' Council of the Arab Countries in the Gulf was established in 1976. The council is composed of six member countries: the United Arab Emirates, Bahrain, Saudi Arabia, Oman, Qatar, and Kuwait. Iraq was also a founding member—however, after Iraq's invasion of Kuwait, Iraq ceased to be a member of the GCC. Later, the Republic of Yemen was invited to join. The council aims to unify the efforts of its members (the Cooperation Council States), strengthening the brotherly ties among them for development of the health services and achieving the highest possible standards of health for the citizens of the council members.

The Health Ministers' Council, together with its Executive Board, is considered a specialized technical organization of the Cooperation Council States, which is geared toward realizing the necessary cooperation and integration among the Cooperation Council States in the various fields of health.

The council includes the Executive Board, which is located in Riyadh. The Executive Board is formed of representative members from all the council states. Each state has one vote, and it is headed by the director general. The Executive Board is the technical, financial, and administrative apparatus, which coordinates and follows up the process of implementation of the health ministers' resolutions and recommendations. It consists of the director general and the technical, financial, and administrative apparatus required to perform its work. Programs of the Executive Board involve more than forty efforts in various fields of health.

---

tourism sector. Higher education benefited from legislative support, norms, and standards from the region's ministries of health in order to improve regulation of the private sector.

During the past few decades, the United Nations organizations and the WHO have greatly aided the GCC states in their various endeavors and in order to eradicate some of the infectious diseases that afflicted the people of the region in the 1950s; to support human development and combat maternal and child health in the 1960s; and to increase the quality of the environment and public health. In more recent years, the WHO has been supporting other health initiatives, such as promoting healthier lifestyles and tobacco cessation.

The governance of national healthcare systems remains a public-sector responsibility in the GCC countries, where ministries of health support health protection, and implement essential public health functions, including surveillance systems and the provision of public goods. Other initiatives include immunization, environmental protection, food fortification, and programs for increased food safety.

Table 1.3 **Medical Schools in the GCC**

Country	No. of IMED Listings	No. of HPED Listings
Bahrain	2	3
Kuwait	1	1
Oman	2	2
Qatar	1	1
Saudi Arabia	24	17
United Arab Emirates	5	4
Total	35	28

Source: Data from M. E. Abdalla and R. Ali Suliman, "Overview of Medical Schools in the Eastern Mediterranean Region of the World Health Organization," *Eastern Mediterranean Health Journal* 19, no. 12 (2013).

Note: IMED, *International Medical Education Directory*; HPED, *Health Professions Education Directory*, WHO/EMRO.

Table 1.4 **Physicians in the GCC per 10,000 Population, 1970–2005**

Country	1970	1990	1995	2000	2005	Ratio, 2005/1970
Bahrain	5.5	13.0	11.1	13.2	27.6	5.0
Kuwait	10.0	14.8	17.8	16.0	18.0	1.8
Oman	0.4	8.6	12.0	13.5	17.9	44.8
Qatar	8.3	18.2	14.3	20.1	27.6	3.3
Saudi Arabia	1.0	18.8	16.6	17.1	20.0	20.0
United Arab Emirates	—	17.5	16.8	17.8	16.1	—

Source: Data from N. M. Kronfol, "Historical Development of Health Professions' Education in the Arab World," *Eastern Mediterranean Health Journal* 18, no. 11 (2012).

Ambulatory Care

The GCC countries' ministries of health are responsible for health promotion through a variety of medical care outlets, centers, private clinics, and hospitals, and they offer national screenings to raise awareness and to promote early detection. In the past, child and maternal healthcare—such as immunization, antenatal care, breastfeeding, and family planning—was the focus of mass public education campaigns. As a result of these campaigns, there have been great improvements in maternal and child health, and there is more current emphasis on the general improvement of health—with programs devoted to smoking cessation; to obesity; to healthier lifestyles; and to screenings for breast, cervical, colon, and prostate cancer, and for HIV/AIDS. The MOH also ensures the provision of safe vaccines and immunizations.

The ways in which GCC populations engage with health centers varies from state to state. Although some families register with PHC, despite the longer waiting times and lack of choice regarding practitioners, others prefer to use what are considered to be more modern private clinics despite the higher cost, but which often offer high quality care.[83]

Hospital Care

Most GCC government-owned hospitals have an excellent level of service, tertiary care, training of human resources, and research. Between 1970 and 1995, there was a rapid increase in public hospitals and health centers in all the GCC countries, which greatly improved the availability of healthcare for the whole population (see table 1.5). Oman and Qatar have allowed their public hospitals to operate autonomously in order to improve administration of their operations.

Quality assurance issues and healthcare sector reforms have risen high on the agendas of the GCC governments. Most ministries of health have set about standardizing the quality of healthcare; submit to accreditation of health facilities; and adhere to guidelines for quality assurance and improvement. International accreditation organizations—including the Joint Commission International, the Canadian accreditation commission, and the Australian accreditation commission—all support the GCC's efforts at certification. The WHO's Eastern Mediterranean Regional Office has asked the national systems to support the accreditation of hospitals and medical colleges, and additional efforts are being

Table 1.5   **Healthcare Services per 10,000 Population in the GCC, about 2005**

Country	Physicians	Dentists	Pharmacists	Nurses	Hospital Beds	PHCC
Bahrain	27.6	4.1	8.3	55.0	27.4	0.3
Kuwait	18.0	3.0	2.0	37.0	19.0	0.4
Oman	17.9	1.9	3.1	37.7	21.0	3.7
Qatar	27.6	5.8	12.6	73.8	25.2	2.7
Saudi Arabia	20.0	2.1	3.5	34.6	23.0	0.8
United Arab Emirates	16.1	4.0	5.8	29.1	18.8	4.0

Source: Data from N. M. Kronfol, "Historical Development of Health Professions' Education in the Arab World," *Eastern Mediterranean Health Journal* 18, no. 11 (2012).

Note: PHCC, primary healthcare corporation.

made to establish accreditation standards for PHC centers and diagnostic facilities. For example, using the WHO's EURO PATH model, Oman has recently introduced efforts to measure hospital performance, and to make further improvements regarding hospital management practices.

Long-Term Care and Palliative Care

Although they have not generated the same interest as acute hospitals, long-term hospitals have existed in most countries of the region for a century to serve the needs of the population. Many of these long-term facilities, which were originally devised as sanatoriums, treated tuberculosis, mental illnesses, and patients with special needs. Though some of these institutions continue to treat communicable diseases such as leprosy, there have been major transformations in their use, and many of them are increasingly serving as hospices for palliative care and to support the elderly.

Treatment Abroad

Many patients in the GCC countries have historically opted for treatment abroad. It was not uncommon for patients with complex medical needs—such as cardiac, neurological, oncological, and pediatric surgery—to be sent for treatment abroad, and these endeavors were often facilitated by the government. Especially in the 1960s and 1970s, when regional healthcare systems were still in their infancy, treatment abroad was frequent; in particular, patients were sent to New Delhi, Beirut, Cairo, Paris, and Berlin. Beirut was known as the "Hospital of the Orient," a reputation to which the city continues to aspire. After the September 11, 2001, terrorist attacks against the United States, there was a decrease in the number of GCC citizens seeking treatment in the United States; instead, they opted to travel to Europe and to other destinations including Thailand, Singapore, and Malaysia.

Despite the massive improvements in the quality and quantity of healthcare facilities and provisions in the GCC states, patients still opt for treatment abroad in certain cases, especially for some of the more serious medical conditions that require greater expertise and higher-quality care. The Crown Prince Courts normally pay for citizens' healthcare requirements and treatment abroad, but do not disclose the overall cost. In some instances, in an effort to control the process, the GCC governments have acquired tertiary care hospitals and healthcare centers abroad, including in London, Geneva, and Glasgow. In other cases, visiting consultants are often invited to the region's public and private hospitals to perform elective surgery.

The United Arab Emirates, especially, is investing in its own healthcare institutions, such as Dubai Healthcare City, in order to attract patients from abroad and to become a center for medical tourism. The Abu Dhabi Chamber of Commerce and Industry reports that in 2010 the United Arab Emirates made massive profits, approximately AED 7 billion ($1.9 billion), from medical tourism.

The Utilization of Pharmaceuticals

Some of the GCC countries, especially Saudi Arabia and the United Arab Emirates, are investing in and developing their own locally based pharmaceutical plants to produce generic medications to be used both domestically and for export. Despite their efforts, they are being pressured by the more established corporate pharmaceutical producers, and their operations are suffering from stiff competition from domestic as well as regional plants.

The Private Sector

In most of the GCC countries, the public sector has been dominant historically. However, as these countries have been engaging in reforming their healthcare systems, they have become increasingly open to support from donor countries and international organizations, especially the World Bank, which study the role of the public sector. Though privatization is not an end in itself, it is being promoted as a solution to some of the setbacks and challenges faced by the public sector, and as a means of improving cost-effectiveness, responsiveness, efficiency, and quality.

Healthcare for the Expatriate Population

In many of the GCC countries, some facilities are restricted to the country's citizens, whereas others are reserved for nonnationals and expatriates. Even though the facilities for expatriates are of good overall standard, nationals receive more support from the government regarding healthcare, a dichotomy related to nationality and sociocultural factors that has been raised many times in discussions.[84]

Table 1.6 **Health Expenditures in the GCC**

Country	% Out-of-Pocket Expenditures per THE	THE per Capita (dollars)
Bahrain	22	690
Kuwait	22	680
Oman	10	300
Qatar	18	1,250
Saudi Arabia	5	500
United Arab Emirates	20	780

Source: Data from Abdel Latif, "Aspiring to Build Health Services and Systems Led by Primary Health Care in the Eastern Mediterranean Region," *Eastern Mediterranean Health Journal* 14, special issue, 2008; adapted from bar diagrams.

Note: THE, total health expenditures.

Private Health Expenditures

Many people living in the GCC countries opt to use private healthcare facilities, which play an increasingly important role in funding healthcare through the payments made to them—which include insurance premiums, fees for private physicians, fees for ambulatory care in the public sector, and payments for over-the-counter goods. Expenditures are also required for a variety of goods and services, including prescription drugs in ambulatory settings, dental services, physiotherapy, hearing aids, and eyeglasses. Private expenditures have increased during the past two decades as a share of total expenditures for health, as shown in table 1.6.

SUMMING UP

The GCC countries have made great improvements to their healthcare systems, which are continually increasing in quality and quantity. Overall, the GCC countries offer an excellent network of hospitals and PHC facilities.[85] The role of each facility is well defined, and quality assurance has become a central focus. The improvements made since the 1970s have catapulted the GCC countries' healthcare services into being some of the best in the world—a remarkable achievement that has been accomplished through perseverance, effective governance, and a commitment to health as an essential human right.[86]

NOTES

1. Donald Bosch and Eloise Bosch, *The Doctor and the Teacher: Oman 1955–1970; Memoirs of Dr. Donald and Eloise Bosch* (Muscat: Apex Publishing, 2000).

2. "Health System Profile: Bahrain," Regional Health Systems Observatory, 2007, http://apps.who.int/medicinedocs/documents/s17291e/s17291e.pdf.

3. Ibid.

4. Ibid.

5. World Health Organization, *Country Cooperation Strategy for WHO and the State of Kuwait, 2005–2009* (Geneva: World Health Organization, 2004).

6. Ibid.

7. Christopher S. Grant and Nayil Al-Kindv, "Surgery in Oman," *Archives of Surgery* 140 (2005): 21–25.

8. Donald Bosch, *The American Mission Hospitals in Oman, 1893–1974, 81 Years* (Muscat: Mazoon, 2002); Bosch and Bosch, *Doctor and the Teacher*.

9. Grant and Al-Kindv, "Surgery in Oman."

10. Qatar Country Study Guide, "Health," http://countrystudies.us/persian-gulf-states/72.htm.

11. Ibid.

12. Fahd Mohammed Albejaidi, "Healthcare System in Saudi Arabia: An Analysis of Structure, Total Quality Management and Future Challenges," *Journal of Alternative Perspectives in the Social Sciences* 2, no. 2 (2010): 794–818.

13. Farhad Al-Harthi et al., "Health over a Century," Riyadh, Ministry of Health and ASBAR Centre for Studies Research and Communication, 1999.

14. Mohammed Hassan S. Mufti, *Healthcare Development Strategies in the Kingdom of Saudi Arabia* (New York: Springer, 2000).

15. Ibid.

16. Ibid.

17. B.Papanikalaou, "The Tuberculosis Control Program in Saudi Arabia," World Health Organization, WHO/TB/I0, 1949, 20–23.

18. Y. Al-Mazrou, T. Khoja, and M. Rao, "Health Services in Saudi Arabia," *Healthcare World Wide: Proceedings of the Annual Conference of the Royal College of Physicians of Edinburgh* 25 (1995): 263–66.

19. Mufti, *Healthcare Development Strategies*.

20. "Health System Profile: Bahrain," Regional Health Systems Observatory, 2007.

21. Ibid.

22. Ibid.

23. Arwa Al Rikabi, Arab News (SRPC), "Dr. Ali Fakhro: The Struggle between Consumerist and Knowledge-Based Economies," http://en-maktoob.news.yahoo.com/dr-ali-fakhro-struggle-between-consumerist-knowledge-based-000000564.html.

24. World Health Organization, *Country Cooperation Strategy for WHO and the State of Kuwait 2005–2009*.

25. Gr ant and Al-Kindv, "Surgery in Oman."

26. Arwa Al Rikabi, Arab News (SRPC), "Dr. Ali Fakhro."

27. R. Smith, "Oman: Leaping across the Centuries," *British Medical Journal* 297 (1988): 540–44.

28. Hasan Ali Mohamed (undersecretary for planning, Ministry of Health), Global Medical Forum Middle East, Beirut, May 2004.

29. Batool Al-Muhandis, WHO consultant, "Implementation of the New Nursing Curriculum in the Ministry of Public Health School of Nursing in Qatar," November 1999.

30. *L'Orient Le Jour Newspaper* (Beirut), March 16, 2005.

31. Raghda Shukri, WHO consultant, "Methodology of Curriculum Development in Qatar," September 1997.

32. Aramco Medical Department, *Epidemiology Bulletin*, Dhahran, Saudi Arabia, October 1972, 1–2.

33. B. Jannadi, H. Alshammari, A. Khan, and R. Hussain, "Current Structure and Future Challenges for the Healthcare System in Saudi Arabia," *Asia Pacific Journal of Health Management* 3, no. 1 (2008): 43–50.

34. Ministry of Health, Kingdom of Saudi Arabia, *Health Statistic Book for the Year of 2006* (Riyadh: Ministry of Health, 2006).

35. Jannadi et al., "Current Structure."

36. Government of Dubai," Our History: Delivering Health from the Start," 2017, www.dha.gov.ae/en/Aboutus/Pages/History.aspx.

37. "United Arab Emirates," Country Data, www.country-data.com/cgi-bin/query/r-14210.html.

38. G. M. Hill, A. Z. Muyeed, and J. A. Al-Lawati, "The Mortality and Health Transition in Oman: Patterns and Processes: A Study Commissioned by the Government of Oman, UNICEF Oman Office, and the WHO Regional Office for the Eastern Mediterranean," December 2000.

39. World Health Organization, *The World Health Report 2000: Health Systems—Improving Performance* (Geneva: World Health Organization, 2000).

40. A. G. Hill and L. C. Chen, *Oman's Leap to Good Health: A Summary of Rapid Health Transition in the Sultanate of Oman* (Muscat: World Health Organization, 1996); Sultanate of Oman Ministry of Health, *Communicable Disease Surveillance and Control*, 2nd ed. (Muscat: Ministry of Health, 2005).

41. Sultanate of Oman Ministry of Health, *Annual Health Reports, 1991–2005* (Muscat: Ministry of Health, 1992–2006).

42. Moeness M. Alshishtawy, "Four Decades of Progress: Evolution of the Health System in Oman," *SQU Medical Journal* 10, no. 1 (2010): 12–22.

43. S. S. Ganguly, M. A. Al-Shafaee, J. A. Al-Lawati, P. K. Dutta, and K. K. Duttagupta, "Epidemiological Transition of Some Diseases in Oman: A Situational Analysis," *Eastern Mediterranean Health Journal* 15, no. 1 (January–February 2009): 209–18.

44. Sultanate of Oman Ministry of Health, "Development of Health Services and Healthcare," www.moh. gov.om/nhjnenu.php?tNm=reports/devoihelt.htm.

45. H. S. Al Bulushi and D. J. West Jr., "Health System Reforms and Community Involvement in Oman," *Journal of Health Sciences Management and Public Health* 7 (2006): 16–28.

46. F. Gadalla, *Outlines of the Health Development Programmes of the Fourth Five-Year Plan (1991–1995)* (Muscat: Ministry of Health, 1993); Sultanate of Oman Ministry of Health, *The Fifth Five-Year Plan for Health Development (1996–2000)* (Muscat: Ministry of Health, 1996); Sultanate of Oman Ministry of Health, *The Sixth Five-Year Plan for Health Development (2001–2005)* (Muscat: Ministry of Health, 2001).

47. A. T. Al-Hinai, *The Needs, the Reality and the Future* (Muscat: Medical Specialty Board, 2003).

48. Ritu Lakhtakia, "Health Professions Education in Oman: A Contemporary Perspective," *SQU Medical Journal* 12, no. 4 (November 2012): 12–22.

49. Grant and Al-Kindv, "Surgery in Oman."

50. Ibid.

51. Government of the State of Qatar, Ministry of Foreign Affairs, "Health Services," 2017, www.mofa.gov.qa/en/qatar/history-of-qatar/health.

52. See the website of the Hamad Medical Corporation, www.hmc.org.qa.

53. Government of the State of Qatar, Ministry of Foreign Affairs, "Health Services."

54. See the website of the National Health Insurance Company, www.nhic.qa.

55. S. Walston, Y. Al-Harbi, and B. Al-Omar, "The Changing Face of Healthcare in Saudi Arabia," *Annals of Saudi Medicine* 28, no. 4 (2008): 243–50.

56. E. B.Gallagher, "Modernization and Health Reform in Saudi Arabia," in *Healthcare Reform around the World*, ed. A. C. Twaddle (London: Auburn House, 2002), 181–97.

57. Kingdom of Saudi Arabia Ministry of Planning, "Achievements of the Development Plans (1970–1985)," 1986, 271; Kingdom of Saudi Arabia Ministry of Health, *Annual Health Report* (Riyadh: Ministry of Health, 1998).

58. The other government bodies include referral hospitals (e.g., King Faisal Specialist Hospital and Research Centre), security forces medical services, army forces medical services, National Guard health affairs, Ministry of Higher Education hospitals (teaching hospitals), Aramco hospitals, Royal Commission for Jubail and Yanbu Health Services, School Health Units of the Ministry of Education, and the Red Crescent Society. Z. Sebai, W. Milaat, and A. Al- Zulaiabani, "Healthcare Services in Saudi Arabia: Past, Present and Future," *Saudi Society of Family and Community Medicine* 8, no. 3 (2001): 93–101.

59. Y. Al-Mazrou, "Prologue," in *Principles and Practice of Primary Healthcare* (Riyadh: Saudi Arabia Ministry of Health, 1990), 7–9.

60. World Health Organization, *Saudi Arabia: Country Cooperation Strategy—At a Glance* (Geneva: World Health Organization, 2011), www.who.int/countryfocus/cooperation_strategy/ccsbrief_sau_en.pdf; M. Al-Malki, G. G. Fitzgerald, and M. Clark, "Healthcare System in Saudi Arabia: An Overview," *Eastern Mediterranean Health Journal* 17, no. 10 (October 2011): 784–93.

61. H. A.Alhusaini, *Obstacles to the Efficiency and Performance of Saudi Nurses at the Ministry of Health, Riyadh Region: Analytical Field Study* (in Arabic) (Riyadh: Ministry of Health, 2006).

62. World Health Organization, *Health System Profile: Saudi Arabia* (Riyadh: WHO Eastern Mediterranean Regional Health System Observatory, n.d.).

63. Jannadi et al., "Current Structure," 43–50.

64. "Vision and Tasks of the Council of Health Services in Saudi Arabia" (in Arabic), Council of Health Services, www.chs.gov.sa/COHS/default.aspx.

65. "New Strategy for Health Services in Saudi Arabia" (in Arabic), *Al-Egtisadia*, September 9, 2009.

66. A. Telmesani, R. G. Zaini, and H. O. Ghazi, "Medical Education in Saudi Arabia: A Review of Recent Developments and Future Challenges," *Eastern Mediterranean Health Journal* 17, no. 8 (August 2011): 20.

67. A. Saati, "Privatization of Public Hospitals: Future Vision and Proposed Framework" (in Arabic), *Al-Egtisadia*, December 3, 2003; "New Strategy for Health Services in Saudi Arabia" (in Arabic), *Al-Egtisadia*, September 9, 2009.

68. Walston, Al-Harbi, and Al-Omar, "Changing Face of Healthcare."

69. "Private Sector Steps Up Role in Saudi Healthcare: As the Saudi Government Steps

Up Efforts to Provide Quality Healthcare to Its Citizens, the Move Opens Up a Massive Opportunity for the Private Sector," www.zawya.com/story/Healthcare_investment_upbeat-ZA WYA20140317060520/?weeklynewsletter&zawyaemailmarketing.

70. M. Al-Yousuf, T. M. Akerele, and Y. Y. Al-Mazrou, "Organisation of the Saudi Health System," *Eastern Mediterranean Health Journal* 8, nos. 4–5 (2002).

71. Saudi Arabia Ministry of Health, "Achievements of the Ministry of Health" (in Arabic), www.moh.gov.sa/Ministry/MediaCenter/News/Pages/NEWS-2007-9-24-001.aspx.

72. F. A. Al-Ateeq, "Experience of Saudi Arabia in Operation of Public Hospitals: The Transition from Companies' Operating System to Self-Operating System," paper presented at Conference on Recent Trends in the Management of Private and Public Hospitals in the Arab World, Arab Administrative Development Organisation, Cairo, March 12–14, 2002.

73. M. Soltis, "Summary of a Quality Assurance Program in Saudi Arabia," *Qualifications Review Board* 12, no. 7 (1986): 266.

74. See the website of the King Faisal Specialist Hospital and Research Center, www.kfshrc .edu.sa; and S. Skillicorn, "Quality Assurance: Mirage or Mirror?" *Annals of Saudi Medicine* 7, no. 2 (1987): 89–92.

75. See the website of the Joint Commission on Accreditation of Hospitals, vvww. jointcommissioninternational.org.

76. Al-Abdul Gader and H. Abdullah, *Managing Computer Based Information Systems in Developing Countries: A Cultural Perspective* (Hershey, PA: IDEA Group, 1999).

77. A. H. Naiaz, *Quality of Healthcare: Theory and Practice* (Riyadh: Ministry of Health Press, 2005); A. H. Naiaz, "The Implementation of Quality Programme in General Directorates in Saudi Arabia," *Quality Journal* 1 (2006): 11.

78. See the website of the Central Board of Accreditation for Healthcare Institutions, www .cbahi.org.sa.

79. N. Kronfol, "Perspectives on the Healthcare System of the United Arab Emirates," *Eastern Mediterranean Health Journal* 5, no. 1 (1999): 149–67.

80. H. Al-Hosani, "Health for All in the United Arab Emirates," *Eastern Mediterranean Health Journal* 6, no. 4 (July 2000): 838–40.

81. "The Role of Government in Health Development," *WHO/EMRO*, 53rd RC, July 2006.

82. The Alma-Ata Declaration affirms that "health is . . . a fundamental human right" and that "a main social target of governments, international organizations, and the whole world community in the coming decades should be the attainment by all peoples of the world by the year 2000 of a level of health that will permit them to lead a socially and economically productive life."

83. Abdalla A. Saeed and Mohamed A. Badreldin, "Patients' Perspective on Factors Affecting Utilization of Primary Healthcare Centers in Riyadh, Saudi Arabia," *Saudi Medical Journal* 23, no. 10 (2002): 1237–42.

84. N. M. Shah, M. A. Shah, and J. Behbehani, "Ethnicity, Nationality and Healthcare Accessibility in Kuwait: A Study of Hospital Emergency Room Users," *Health Policy Plan* 11, no. 3 (September 1996): 319–28.

85. Adapted from *WHO EMRO*.

86. "The infant mortality rate in Oman was reduced from 118 per 1,000 live births in 1970 to 10.25 per 1,000 live births in 2008, and the under-5 mortality rate was similarly reduced, from 181 per 1,000 live births in 1970 to 11 per 1,000 live births in 2008" (Abdel Latif).

THE POLITICS OF HEALTHCARE IN THE GULF COOPERATION COUNCIL STATES

Dionysis Markakis

Healthcare constitutes a fundamental concern for most contemporary societies across the world. Advances in healthcare provision during the twentieth century have had a radical impact on human life, contributing significant improvements in both quality and duration. This is clearly illustrated by the fact that in 1900, the average human life span was just thirty-one years. A century later, this figure had more than doubled, to sixty-five years, as of 2005.[1] Accordingly, the provision of healthcare has emerged as one of the basal functions of most competent, modern states—with many citizens positing it in fact as an obligation, a central tenet of the so-called social contract.

This is no less true of the countries in the Gulf region, where healthcare has emerged as a leading issue for both states and societies. In Saudi Arabia, a 2004 poll identified healthcare as the primary concern for the country's citizens, with political participation notably coming far lower. A similar result was also found in the United Arab Emirates.[2] This evinces one of the many nuances characteristic of the Gulf states, whereby untaxed citizenries are ruled by unrepresentative governments, which nonetheless bestow many of the benefits of the modern state apparatus on their respective populations. Healthcare in particular is one such area, with the Gulf region currently witnessing record levels of investment. In 2015 the Gulf Cooperation Council (GCC) healthcare market was worth $43.9 billion, a rise of 11 percent annually from 2010, when it stood at $25.6 billion.[3] This can be seen in contrast to the typical, monodimensional depictions of authoritarian rule, whereby the relationship between ruler and ruled is portrayed predominantly as one of repression and exploitation.

This chapter examines the politics of healthcare in the context of the Gulf, limited here to the GCC member countries. It argues that healthcare constitutes an intrinsic component of the tacit social contract between the Gulf region's ruling families and their respective citizenries. In return for citizens' loyalty, the ruling families provide a wide range of social welfare benefits gratis, including employment, education, and healthcare. First, the chapter analyzes the introduction of modern healthcare in the Gulf region. Second, it examines the contextual parameters—namely, the main issues that have an impact on healthcare provision (e.g., the endemic obesity rates among the region's citizens). Third, it explores the role healthcare assumes in the Gulf region's social contract, deconstructing what the provision of healthcare in the Gulf means in political terms. Fourth and finally, it addresses the main challenges faced by the Gulf states in their attempts to create sustainable healthcare infrastructures.

MODERN HEALTHCARE IN THE GULF REGION

The emergence of modern healthcare infrastructures in the countries of the GCC mirror broader historical trends in the region. The transformation of healthcare in the Gulf region became evident in the twentieth century, with Bahrain and Kuwait, under the guidance of Western religious missionaries, being among the first Gulf countries to open public hospitals. The close interactions with the British Empire also had an impact on the development of healthcare in the region. For instance, Oman's long-standing relationship with Britain, as a key commercial trading post on the route to colonial-era India, resulted in the British Consulate funding the first Omani hospital in 1910. This was also the case in the United Arab Emirates, known then as the Trucial Coast due to the various sheikhdoms' treaties with the British, which led to the building of a public hospital in Dubai, although this came relatively late, in 1949. In contrast to the other Gulf states, however, Saudi Arabia had a more insular experience, which resulted in organized healthcare developing considerably later.[4]

Given that these developments took place alongside the expansion of European influence in the region, one needs to consider the underlying political context—namely, the role assumed by healthcare in colonial administration systems.[5] Hubert Lyautey, a French army general and colonial administrator known as the "Maker of Morocco," was one of the early proponents of incorporating healthcare into colonial ventures. He told his commanding officer during France's efforts to pacify Madagascar in 1901 that "if you can send me four doctors, I will send you back four companies."[6] Lyautey later claimed that "colonial expansion has its harsh aspects, . . . [but] if there is something that ennobles it and justifies it, it is the action of the doctor, understood as a mission and an apostleship."[7] The roots of modern healthcare in the Gulf therefore lie in the colonial era. Colonialism was viewed on one hand as a means of pacifying local populations and ensuring their cooperation, and on the other hand as a way of "civilizing" them, by introducing them to Western practices.[8] This has broad parallels today in terms of state–society relations in the Gulf, whose ruling families have positioned the provision of healthcare as a key means of ensuring their citizens' loyalty but also as a central feature of the processes of state modernization under way. It is also worth noting that the Gulf states' colonial legacies entailed the introduction of a very specific conception of healthcare and its application, one rooted in a quite different context from the Gulf. This rings particularly true in the contemporary GCC countries, when one considers the ongoing wholesale importing of healthcare knowledge from the West. It raises questions about the one-sided nature of this interaction, and it feeds into broader debates about core–periphery relations. The implications of this mode of importation, and whether it is sensible and indeed sustainable, are explored further below.

Since the Gulf states attained independence in the 1960s and 1970s, the regional healthcare infrastructure has developed rapidly, on a largely unprecedented scale in global terms. This has been made possible through two related factors, which are characteristic of the Gulf states. The first is the centralized, monopolized form of power that is practiced, and the second is the rentier nature of these economies. This has had a unique impact on the scope, depth, and pace of state development in the Gulf in general, and correspondingly also in terms of healthcare. Over the last forty years or so, the vast proceeds of hydrocarbon extraction, combined with the largely uncontested visions of development outlined by the Gulf monarchies, has fueled the growth of the healthcare industry. Saudi Arabia, for instance, opened about eighty hospitals in the period from 1970 to 1985.[9] By the end of 1990, this number had increased to more than 250 facilities.[10] In 2010 a total of 415 hospitals, both governmental and private, existed.[11] Another example is Oman, which in 1970 had only two hospitals in the entire country. But in 2000 the World Health Organization (WHO) ranked Oman first in healthcare delivery efficiency and utilization of financial resources among 191 countries, while also featuring it in the top ten of the world's most effective healthcare systems overall.[12]

This reflects a panregional trend in healthcare. Driven by high levels of state investment, and grounded in collaborations with a range of established international institutions—including Harvard University, Imperial College London, Johns Hopkins University, and Weill Cornell Medicine, among others—an attempt to construct a potentially exemplary healthcare infrastructure is being made in the Gulf region.[13] In 2010 Suzanne Robertson-Malt noted that "there are a total of 132 hospital projects under way in the GCC with a combined construction value of US$17,917 million. The three largest projects under development are Sidra Medical & Research Center, Doha, Qatar (US$2,300 million); Jaber Al Ahmed Al Sabah Hospital, Surra, Kuwait (US$1,200 million); and 2,000 health clinics throughout Saudi Arabia (US$1,000 million)."[14]

As a result of these processes of development in recent decades, the Gulf region currently boasts some of the highest life-expectancy rates in the Middle East, in terms of national citizens. It also has some of the lowest regional infant mortality rates.[15] In concrete terms, from 1978 to 2004, life expectancy across the GCC rose from sixty to seventy-three years, while infant mortality fell from 69 deaths per 1,000 live births to a relatively low 18.[16] By 2010 infant mortality had fallen to 13, while life expectancy had reached an average of almost seventy-five years.[17] And though contagious diseases such as malaria and measles were once prevalent in the region, they have largely been eliminated today.[18]

HEALTHCARE IN THE GULF REGION: CONTEXTUAL PARAMETERS

The expansion of healthcare has not been motivated solely by the largesse of the Gulf region's ruling families. In practice, it has emerged in large part through necessity. It is perhaps ironic that many of the diseases that feature in the contemporary region are the products of the very affluence afforded by its vast hydrocarbon revenues. The rapid onset of modernization, or perhaps more accurately Westernization, has had a direct and measurable impact on the region's societies, introducing fundamentally unhealthy lifestyles.[19] As a result, the GCC countries currently constitute "one of the most obese regions in the world," with about 40 percent of its national citizens classified as such.[20] This is in line with trends in the broader Middle East, where about two-thirds of the adult population are classified as overweight.[21] These trends are manifested primarily in a range of noncommunicable diseases, such as heart attacks, strokes, cancer, diabetes, and asthma.[22] For instance, a 2014 study found that more than 66 percent of male and 60 percent of female citizens of the United Arab Emirates were either overweight or obese.[23] This is true of the Gulf region as a whole, where obesity and the related type 2 diabetes are prevalent at a much higher rate than anywhere else in the world.[24]

This situation is compounded by three broader contextual factors, which are having a significant impact on healthcare policy in the Gulf and will increasingly do so in the near future. The first factor is population growth, which currently lies at 3 percent annually across the region, one of the highest rates in the world. As a measure of comparison, it is estimated that by 2025 the total population of the GCC will nearly double in size, predominantly due to immigration.[25] The extremely high percentage of expatriates residing within most GCC countries, and the rapid rate at which these populations are increasing, inevitably has an impact on healthcare delivery in the region. For instance, the population of Qatar is estimated to have nearly doubled since 2007, with commensurate burdens placed on infrastructure, education, and healthcare.[26]

The second factor is the fact that improvements in life expectancy and infant mortality reduction have led to significant increases in the number of national citizens in the Gulf over the age of sixty-five years. In Saudi Arabia alone, this demographic is expected to increase sevenfold over the next twenty-five years.[27] In Oman, a sixfold increase is anticipated.[28] In other words, the population of the Gulf region is growing rapidly, with the average citizen living far longer, yet the region's societies are facing a host of health challenges, associated in large part with the processes of modernization that are under way. This has clear implications for the sustainability of the region's established social contract.

The third factor is the high level of urbanization and development in the region. Approximately 80 percent of Gulf residents live in highly concentrated metropolitan areas, which, for example, have associated effects on health, through pollution. This is compounded by the stratified nature of the Gulf region's cities, with national citizens and white-collar expatriates living in conditions of relative luxury, in contrast to blue-collar manual laborers, the majority of whom live in far less equitable conditions, with significant associated effects on quality of life. The latter, as Maria Kristiansen and Aziz Sheikh note,

> tend to be employed as construction workers, domestic helpers, cleaners, and drivers—jobs characterized by low payment, long working hours, and, at times, physically and mentally hazardous working conditions. Furthermore, many of these migrants experience poor housing conditions and have limited access to quality healthcare. These factors result in a number of adverse health outcomes, including high rates of work-related

accidents and mental health problems. Gross human rights violations—including human trafficking, mental abuse, and sexual and other physical violence—sometimes compound these health risks.[29]

It is important here to highlight a fact that is often overlooked in statistics addressing the Gulf region—namely, that the figures cited apply exclusively to national citizens, thus excluding expatriate residents, who in fact constitute the majority of most GCC countries' populations, with the exceptions of Saudi Arabia and Oman.[30] This is particularly relevant in terms of health-related figures. For instance, the obesity endemic in the Gulf concerns predominantly national citizens, and thus a minority of the overall population. This has significant implications for the formulation and implementation of healthcare policies in the region, given the fact that the citizens' healthcare needs differ considerably from those of expatriate residents; and this is particularly true when one distinguishes between white-collar and blue-collar laborers. Thus, the healthcare infrastructures of the Gulf region's states need to address at least three distinct populations, each with very different needs and requirements. This can be seen in the case of Qatar, where upon arrival all expatriate workers are medically screened for a range of diseases, including for tuberculosis, a disease that has been largely eradicated from the developed world but is prevalent in the countries where most laborers originate. In fact, migrant workers from countries such as Nepal, India, and the Philippines are required to also undergo these tests before arrival, in contrast to expatriates arriving from Western countries such as the United States and the United Kingdom.[31] This illustrates the diverse, complex needs of the various populations that Gulf healthcare infrastructures address.

HEALTHCARE: A PILLAR OF THE GULF SOCIAL CONTRACT

At its heart, healthcare is a fundamentally political issue. In most societies, access to healthcare provision, and the quality thereof, is determined by a number of factors, including race, class, and gender. In the context of the Gulf, this has a crucial added dimension, given that healthcare constitutes a fundamental component of the ruling families' strategies of co-option. Citizenship in the Gulf region is largely based on social welfare entitlements, with the provision of healthcare, and other such benefits, serving as a means of ensuring that citizens remain dependent on the state, and therefore politically quiescent. As Ahmed al-Mukhaini, a former adviser to Oman's Shura Council, rationalized: "If you want to enjoy the perks, you have to abide by certain regulations. If you want to be my citizen, keep quiet."[32]

Healthcare can be seen as one of a range of tools at the disposal of authoritarian regimes, which incorporate "soft" facets, such as healthcare and education, as well as "hard" facets, such as violence and repression. One of the many examples in the Gulf region was Iraq during the 1980s, which combined one of the most advanced healthcare systems in the region with one of the most repressive political systems. This multifaceted approach is characteristic of other contemporary GCC countries.

Beyond this, one needs to consider the broader patriarchal dynamics that underpin governance in the Gulf region. Michael Hudson argues: "Patrimonial respect is the rule. The tradition of patrimonial deference extends beyond the family itself to the people who, in the ideal case, submit themselves as a flock unto a shepherd."[33] The head of the ruling family is positioned, by extension, as the father of the nation; as such, the onus to serve as provider to the people follows. This patriarchal framework derives from the central role assumed by the tribe in Gulf region politics, on whose extensive, intertwined familial networks the contemporary Gulf states are built. As a result, tribal allegiance constitutes one of the primary sources of any Gulf ruler's legitimacy. This allegiance is secured in large part through the provision of benefits, such as healthcare, framed as a benevolent exchange from the ruler to the people.

The maintenance of the social contract in the Gulf region constitutes a perpetual challenge for the various ruling families. This is seen in terms of ensuring stability, and, most important, the continuity of their monopolized form of rule. The delicate nature of this bargain is illustrated by the example of Bahrain, whose dwindling oil resources prefaced an abrogation of the social contract, culminating in a popular uprising against the monarchy in 2011. The protests were driven in no small part by the ruling Al-Khalifa family's failure to provide satisfactory employment, education, and healthcare to significant portions of its citizenry. Although these were clearly not the only variables—with sectarian divisions also being relevant, for example—the decaying social welfare system constituted a central grievance for protestors. With tensions ongoing, Bahrain points toward the inherent fragility of the social contract in the Gulf, although it is worth noting that this is more relevant in the cases of Oman or Saudi Arabia, than, say, Qatar or the United Arab Emirates.

The Gulf ruling families clearly comprehend the vital importance healthcare assumes in the social contract. In this respect the Gulf states can be clearly differentiated from other countries in the Middle East, say, Lebanon or Egypt, where nonstate actors such as Hezbollah and the Muslim Brotherhood have assumed important roles in social welfare provision, including healthcare, due to the weaknesses of the state itself. For instance, Shawn Teresa Flanigan and Mounah Abdel-Samad note in the case of Hezbollah that its Islamic Health Unit performs "a vital function in meeting public health needs. It operates three hospitals, 12 health centers, 20 infirmaries, 20 dental clinics, and 10 defense departments. The Islamic Health unit has been so effective that it was asked to assume the operation of several government hospitals in Southern Lebanon and the Bekaa Valley. . . . [It] provides healthcare to low-income Shiites and other low-income populations at little or no cost."[34] For such nonstate actors, the provision of social welfare services has constituted an important means of garnering popular support and legitimacy.

Strong public administration on the part of the Gulf states has prevented this from taking place there, in no small measure because of the ruling families' recognition of the incipient threat. This applies to nongovernmental organizations more generally, domestic and foreign, which remain severely circumscribed in the Gulf. The current trend of advocating for the introduction of privatized healthcare models in the Gulf—this on the part of a range of international consultancies including McKinsey, Booz Allen Hamilton, and Alpen Capital—therefore seemingly underestimates the nuanced role healthcare assumes in the Gulf social contract.[35] Although the Gulf states do utilize bilateral partnerships with international organizations—Abu Dhabi's Cleveland Eye Clinic is one example—the state retains a high degree of involvement in these initiatives, and subsequently overall control. Perhaps most importantly, the state adopts a highly visible role in such "public–private" partnerships—in the case of the Cleveland Eye Clinic, by framing it as an initiative of the state-led Mubadala Development company.[36] This means that the state is clearly positioned as the provider to the people, munificently upholding its side of the social contract.

The approach to healthcare provision in the Gulf is characteristic of policy formulation and implementation as a whole, which is inherently top-down in nature. Alongside the concerted effort to restrict substantive manifestations of civil society, this arguably has negative effects on policy implementation, not least healthcare. Monopolized by the state, with a lack of input from independent civil society actors, healthcare policy can often appear arbitrary and ad hoc. In no small part, this is because of the relative absence of civil society, one of whose basic functions is to convey citizens' perspectives on government policy in an organized, coherent manner.[37] This is exacerbated by an overwhelming reliance on foreign consultancies to design and implement healthcare policies in the region, which more likely than not results in the underutilization, if not exclusion, of relevant local knowledge and participation.[38]

The Gulf ruling families' comprehension of healthcare's vital importance in the social contract is reflected in the fact that a substantial percentage of Gulf citizens seek medical treatment abroad, even for relatively minor ailments, with the costs borne by the state. In 2009 alone, the United Arab Emirates spent $2 billion on medical treatment for citizens abroad.[39] Jay Loschky of Gallup argues: "Sizable numbers of nationals in Gulf Cooperation Council countries say they would prefer to seek medical attention outside of their own country if they had a serious health concern. Among the GCC nationals surveyed in 2011, Kuwaitis (65 percent) are the most likely to prefer to receive medical care abroad, and Saudis (35 percent) are the least likely."[40] This raises questions regarding the impact of this outsourcing on trust levels between Gulf citizens and their respective governments, and correspondingly, if this has any effect on the popular standing or legitimacy of the ruling families in the Gulf. A 2010 poll on citizens' life evaluations across the GCC found a large breadth of responses:

> Life evaluations are highest in the UAE [United Arab Emirates], where about two-thirds of nationals are classified as thriving. Life evaluations are lowest in Bahrain, where slightly more than one-quarter of nationals fall into the [economic] thriving category. . . . In Qatar, 56 percent of nationals are classified as thriving, while 42 percent fall into the [economic] struggling category. Thriving and struggling are split in Saudi Arabia, 43 percent and 52 percent, respectively. A slight majority of nationals in Kuwait are classified as struggling, while 44 percent are thriving.[41]

The relatively high numbers of Gulf citizens who identify as struggling—typically a correlate of factors such as income, education, and health—hints toward some of the potential underlying challenges faced by the GCC countries.

This has spurred efforts to develop high-standard, comprehensive healthcare infrastructures within the region. Abdulla Abdul Aziz Al-Shamsi, executive administrative officer of the Cleveland Clinic in Abu Dhabi, claims: "There is a lot of money that is spent by the government on providing care for UAE nationals, specifically providing care for them abroad. . . . The opportunity . . . is to reinstate that care back as an option here in Abu Dhabi, and this relationship is allowing us to be able to deliver that healthcare, but also create something that has never been done anywhere around the world."[42] The United Arab Emirates also features two healthcare "free zones," Dubai Healthcare City and Dubai Biotechnology and Research Park.[43] The former is one of the largest regional healthcare destinations, attracting about ten-thousand visitors in 2011, as part of a nascent medical tourism sector.[44]

Such projects form a crucial part of the broader state-building efforts embarked on by the various ruling families of the Gulf region, ranging from education to infrastructure, to modernize and develop their societies and create sustainable economies beyond rentierism. As such, healthcare constitutes a key facet of the modern, knowledge-based economies envisioned by the Gulf region's ruling families. This is reflected in the attempts to introduce medical research cultures in the region. Saudi Arabia signed an agreement with the highly respected *British Medical Journal* for cooperation in "health learning and research"—for instance, as part of a "20-year workforce transformation strategy to improve the consistency and quality of healthcare across the Kingdom."[45] In a similar vein, Qatar's National Research Fund has committed about 24 percent of its budget to research on noncommunicable diseases.[46] One such project is Weill Cornell Medicine–Qatar's mapping of the native Qatari DNA genome in an attempt to address inherited diseases prevalent in the local population of nationals.[47] Whether in Dubai or Abu Dhabi or Doha, the realization that hydrocarbon resources are ultimately finite has spurred an effort, still in its early stages, to construct innovative, competitive national economies. Not least, the intention is to provide employment opportunities for national citizens. For instance, in 2013 Oman announced the construction of a $1.5 billion medical complex to be located in Batinah, one of the focal points of popular unrest in 2011.[48] The development of healthcare, whether in infrastructural or research terms, subsequently constitutes an integral aspect of the Gulf states' political visions.

These activities feed into broader discussions of healthcare as part of the social contract—namely, its role as a public good. For instance, the WHO defines health as "a state of complete physical, mental and social well-being and not merely the absence of disease or infirmity."[49] This is referenced by the *Lancet*, which posits healthcare as a basic human right: "The provision of universal healthcare in all Gulf countries should be mandatory: health is a human right, and the rights of all patients to both treatment and psychosocial support are paramount. The disproportionate distribution of wealth in the region is a substantial hurdle to accessing care for a large part of the population, which hinders efforts toward universal care."[50] The latter refers to the vast numbers of manual laborers who, despite implementing the visions of development articulated by the Gulf states, lack many of the rights of other white-collar expatriates, let alone citizens—perhaps most pressingly in terms of healthcare. Such workers' access to healthcare is dependent on their employers, with predictable conflicts of interest arising.[51] Additionally, some workers are brought in to work illicitly on temporary tourist visas, and without residency permits cannot access the national healthcare systems. This of course concerns basic healthcare. If one adopts the WHO's more holistic definition of healthcare articulated above, then the inequality of healthcare access across the Gulf region becomes even more pronounced.

The equity of healthcare access is a central issue. Although, on the surface, this primarily concerns manual laborers, who are by definition temporary residents of the countries concerned, it also affects other more permanent, marginalized groups in the Gulf region. One notable example is the Bidoon in Kuwait, residents within Kuwait but lacking citizenship, who are subsequently denied the benefits of the welfare state. For instance, since 1993 the Bidoon have been required to pay for access to basic healthcare services. In 2006 an exemption was granted for those under the age of eighteen years and those deemed handicapped.[52] Numbering about 100,000 in total, the primary reason for their exclusion by the state is to restrict the numbers of those with access to social welfare benefits. Although Kuwait has the largest number of Bidoon, they are present in most of the GCC countries.[53] Another group, albeit much smaller, increasingly affected in the region are those nationals whose citizenship is revoked, predominantly for political reasons. This has occurred in Kuwait, Bahrain, and the United Arab Emirates—the intended purpose being to disenfranchise political opponents completely. Hamad al-Bloshi, a professor at Kuwait University, argues: "The issue of citizenship in Kuwait—it's life. . . . Your work, your home, your children's school, your health, your car, . . . all these things, they can take from you."[54] This reflects the intrinsic role that social welfare benefits, including healthcare, assume in the unwritten social contract between state and citizens in the Gulf. It underscores that healthcare is fundamentally political in nature, and perhaps more so in the context of the Gulf than elsewhere.

The issue of equity is also relevant on a broader level, in terms of gender. This is true of the Gulf region but also of the wider Middle East, with reference to the regressive gender roles perpetuated by societies across the region. In terms of healthcare, this is particularly pressing with regard to women's sexual and reproductive health. Thoraya Ahmed Obaid, executive director of the United Nations Population Fund, argues:

Reproductive health is not merely an individual matter; it is a matter that involves the community and the society. Why? Because these issues touch on issues of culture and religion, and they touch on values, traditions, and practices. They also touch the traditional patriarchal structures in the communities—structures that establish and maintain power relations between women and men and among the community at large. And that is why improving reproductive health requires improvement in the status of women as one of the basic human rights.[55]

As the largest constituency of healthcare recipients, due to reproduction, women in the Gulf region have remarkably little say in healthcare policy formulation and implementation. This is a direct reflection of the patriarchal societal structure that they inhabit.[56] As Farzaneh Roudi-Fahimi, director of the Middle East and North Africa (MENA) Program at the Population Reference Bureau, notes: "A pervasive culture of silence influences the way MENA women perceive their bodies and their health. And this culture also circumscribes their 'health-seeking behaviors'—whether and where they look for health services."[57]

HEALTHCARE IN THE GULF REGION: A SUSTAINABLE MODEL?

A central tenet of the social contract, and a key feature of the state-building processes under way, healthcare policy in the Gulf region faces a number of important challenges. As Mona Mourshed and colleagues note: "[The GCC countries] will face an unparalleled and unprecedented rise in demand for healthcare over the course of the next two decades. . . . No other region in the world faces such rapid growth in demand with the simultaneous need to realign its healthcare systems to be able to treat the disorders of affluence."[58] Aside from the contextual parameters discussed above—namely, the Gulf's unhealthy, aging, and growing population, living amid rapid urbanization and development—there are a number of questions regarding the overall sustainability of healthcare policy in the Gulf, and subsequently its role in the social contract. The challenges faced by healthcare policy in the Gulf derive from broader trends in the Gulf states, which are by and large exceptional—in political, economic, and social terms. The processes of state formation, the rapid pace of development, the resources on which these states are being built, and the skewed demographics necessitated all constitute a unique experiment in contemporary state building. This has resulted in a number of equally unique challenges.

The first challenge is the economic sustainability of the healthcare model in question. Traditionally, in high-income countries healthcare is financed through taxation, whereas in low-income countries, external sources such as foreign aid are key.[59] In this sense, the GCC countries can be distinguished from both high- and low-income countries. The question of sustainability arises with regard to the limited role assumed by the private sector. Across the region, state expenditures dominate healthcare budgets, with the private sector assuming a by far subsidiary role.[60] This model is ultimately sustainable only as long as hydrocarbon revenues accrue to high levels—which, given abrupt fluctuations in prices, and, moreover, the finite nature of the resource—remains a tenuous chance at best. To address this challenge, in the face of disproportionate expatriate populations, the GCC countries have sought to minimize the financial burden on the state, increasingly passing the cost of noncitizens' healthcare on to employers. The proportion of nongovernmental healthcare expenditures as a proportion of total healthcare expenses in GCC countries ranges from 18 to 33 percent. This is reflected in Abu Dhabi, whose staggered introduction of mandatory health insurance for all residents, as part of a wide-ranging healthcare reform initiative, is generally regarded as a progressive model in the regional context. Abu Dhabi instituted a three tiered insurance system, addressing the distinct populations that make up the Gulf states, as discussed above. National citizens, more than 400,000 individuals, are insured under the "Thiqa" (Trust) cover. This provides comprehensive, complementary coverage by the state, and extends well beyond basic physical health to include generous allowances for mental healthcare, dietary consultations, home care, and so forth.[61] White-collar expatriate workers, numbering more than 1 million in total, are insured under the "Enhanced" cover, which is paid by their respective employers. And finally, blue-collar workers, or those earning under $1,000 per month, numbering over 1.3 million in total, are insured under the "Basic" cover, which is again financed by the employer.

Unlike Thiqa, those covered under the Enhanced and Basic covers need to make copayments, primarily for medication and for optical and dental services.[62] Erik Koornneef and colleagues note that "there are noticeable differences in the utilization of healthcare between different groups as reflected in the percentage of claims per health scheme: 15.7 percent of insured individuals hold a Thiqa card, compared with 47 percent who have Basic insurance. However, as a percentage of the amount claimed, Thiqa card holders represent 40.1 percent of the market, whereas Basic insurance card holders represent 26.5 percent."[63] The discrepancies in the rates of healthcare utilization can be attributed to the fact that those insured under Basic plans are predominantly young, expatriate males, who are by definition transient. Those covered under Thiqa plans include women and those over the retirement age of sixty-five, constituencies that tend to have higher healthcare needs. Also, one needs to consider the prevalence of lifestyle diseases among the nationals who make up the Thiqa plan holders. A final consideration is the fact that those on Basic insurance need to make a higher level of copayment.[64] Abu Dhabi's tiered healthcare insurance policy reflects the segregated demography of the Gulf states. It raises questions about the issues of equity discussed above, particularly when contrasted with other national healthcare systems. One example is the United Kingdom's National Health Service, a cornerstone of the country's post–World War II social contract, which provides free, equitable access to all residents alike, regardless of citizenship.

The second challenge to the sustainability of the healthcare model in the Gulf region again derives from the region's demographic composition—namely, the high distribution of expatriates, which is acutely reflected in the healthcare industry. Healthcare professionals in the Gulf region are overwhelmingly expatriates and by definition transient, with shortages of qualified staff, amid high turnover rates, a pressing issue throughout the region. This has clear implications for the sustainability of healthcare in the Gulf region: "Currently around 20 qualified physicians serve every 10,000 people, compared to approximately 27 doctors in the US and UK systems indicating a shortage of about 180,000 specialists. According to WHO, the MENA region [as a whole] has 3.5 dentistry staff and 28.4 nurses per 10,000 people, which is nearly 79 percent and 71 percent respectively lower compared to the US."[65] One of the inherent weaknesses of the healthcare model in the region is that as a result of this reliance on expatriates, medical professionals are sourced from a range of different backgrounds, with a commensurate range of qualifications, and therefore capabilities. This has encouraged the emergence of varying healthcare standards: "Health workers are migrating to the Gulf from both developed and developing nations, breaking the conception of North and South as destination and source. A two-tier system is emerging, where health worker migrants to the GCC who are 'Western trained' are valued higher, compensated better, placed in urban centers, granted more senior positions, and have greater opportunities/ training available."[66] One of the attempts to address this expatriate dependency is under way in Oman, where the policy of "Omanization" introduced in the 1990s has led to the creation of an accredited national medical university, and increased levels of qualified Omani medical personnel.[67] This reflects a growing trend in the region, with a total of twenty-seven medical colleges formed across the Gulf, the majority in Saudi Arabia, which has a total of sixteen; followed by the United Arab Emirates, with five; Bahrain and Oman, with two each; and Kuwait and Qatar, with one each.[68]

Overall, the GCC countries have undertaken a concerted effort to address the underlying weaknesses of the regional healthcare infrastructure, manifested in record levels of investment. Although many of the challenges they face are common to the region, each country has largely forged its own path. For example, Saudi Arabia—the largest healthcare market in the region, accounting for about 46 percent of the total GCC market—introduced a healthcare budget of approximately $29 billion in 2014.[69] With one of the most developed healthcare infrastructures in the Middle East, in comparison with Western countries it still suffers from chronic shortages of medical staff and hospital beds.[70] By comparison, one of the smallest regional healthcare markets, Qatar, is the highest per capita healthcare spender in the GCC and the broader Middle East.[71] In 2012 Qatar spent more than $4 billion on healthcare.[72] Qatar's Supreme Council of Health claimed: "This represents an increase of 25 percent since 2011, and 64 percent since 2009; . . . [at $2,270,] Qatar's per capita THE [total health expenditures] was higher than the GCC average, at US $1,251, but lower than the OECD [Organization for Economic Cooperation and Development] average, at US $3,354."[73] Perhaps as a result of this, a poll by Gallup in the GCC found that "Qatar had the highest levels of [healthcare] satisfaction, at 90 percent, followed by the UAE, at 79 percent." Kuwait and Saudi Arabia came last.[74]

Yet as a whole, the GCC countries' investment in healthcare remains relatively low compared with the OECD countries' spending—considerably less than half per capita on average, at $1,251, compared with $3,354.[75] Bassam Ramadan, the World Bank's country manager in Kuwait, states that "[GCC] government spending on healthcare remains low and does not meet people's expectations. . . . The GCC governments spend an average of 7 percent of their annual budgets on healthcare compared to the 17 percent spent by OECD countries."[76] But ultimately, addressing the underlying issues concerning healthcare in the GCC requires more than mere financial investment. Enis Baris, the World Bank's sector manager for health in the MENA region, called for a comprehensive strategy: "Revisiting the values and principles that underpin health systems for more pluralistic and accountable health system governance. In the GCC countries this would mean rethinking the way healthcare is financed and organized to align incentives for improved access to, and continuity of, appropriate care in primary care settings. It also means reaching out to other sectors to set up the regulatory framework for tobacco control, or prevention of road injuries."[77]

The issues that the GCC states need to address are long term and complex, and range from healthier lifestyle choices, to more balanced urban planning, to the development of sustainable workforces of nationals. Many of these concern broader social, economic, and political issues, which are related to the unique processes of state building under way in the Gulf region, amid rapid growth and modernization. As such, the solutions to these issues remain elusive.

NOTES

1. Thomson Prentice, "Health, History and Hard Choices: Funding Dilemmas in a Fast-Changing World," *WHO's Global Health Histories*, August 2006, www.who.int/global_health_histories/seminars/presentation07.pdf.

2. James Zogby, *Attitudes of Arabs: An In-Depth Look at Social and Political Concerns of Arabs* (Washington, DC: Arab American Institute and Zogby International, 2005), 6.

3. Isaac John, "GCC Healthcare Market to Hit $44 Billion Mark by 2015," *Khaleej Times*, October 2, 2013, www.khaleejtimes.com/kt-article-display-1.asp?section=uaebusiness&xfile=data/uaebusiness/2013/october/uaebusiness_october21.xml.

4. See chapter 1 in this volume, by Nabil M. Kronfol.

5. Joe Stork, "Political Aspects of Health," *Middle East Review* 19 (1989), www.merip.org/mer/mer161/political-aspects-health?ip_login_no_cache=fdf3364b9c6378bec9ba6e3921b8b225.

6. Ibid.

7. Ibid.

8. Cynthia Myntti, "Medical Education: The Struggle for Relevance," *Middle East Review* 19 (1989), www.merip.org/mer/mer161/medical-education-struggle-relevance.

9. Stork, "Political Aspects of Health."

10. Ibid.

11. Ministry of Health, *Statistical Book* (Riyadh: Saudi Ministry of Health, 2010), www.moh.gov.sa/en/Ministry/Statistics/book/Pages/default.aspx.

12. "New Challenges to the Healthcare System in Oman," Oman Information Center, www.omaninfo.com/health/new-challenges-healthcare-system-oman.asp.

13. Suzanne Robertson-Malt, "Cultural Intelligence and the Delivery of Healthcare in the GCC Countries," *Avicenna* 1 (2010): 1.

14. Ibid.

15. "World Population Prospects: The 2012 Revision," United Nations Development Program, 2013, http://esa.un.org/wpp/documentation/pdf/wpp2012_highlights.pdf.

16. Mona Mourshed, Viktor Hediger, and Toby Lambert, *Gulf Cooperation Council Health Care: Challenges and Opportunities*, McKinsey Global Competitiveness Reports (New York: McKinsey & Company, 2006), 56, www.weforum.org/pdf/Global_Competitiveness_Reports/Reports/chapters/2_1.pdf.

17. United Nations Development Program, *Human Development Report, 1980–2013* (New

York: United Nations, 2014), http://knoema.com/HDR2013/human-development-report
-1980-2012?location=1002130-gcc.

18. Mourshed, Hediger, and Lambert, *Gulf Cooperation Council Health Care*, 56.

19. Informa Exhibitions, "Healthcare in the GCC: A Snapshot," *Hospital Build &
Infrastructure Magazine* 3 (2012): 11, http://inc.informa-mea.com/Sites/HospitalBuild/v1
/Downloads/resources/articles/Regional%20healthcare/regional_healthcare.pdf.

20. Ibid.; Mourshed, Hediger, and Lambert, *Gulf Cooperation Council Health Care*, 56.

21. Informa Exhibitions, "Healthcare in the GCC," 11.

22. See "Noncommunicable Diseases," WHO Fact Sheet, January 2015, www.who.int
/mediacentre/factsheets/fs355/en.

23. Lindsay Carroll, "Obesity in the Gulf: Disturbing New Survey," *The National*, May 29,
2014, www.thenational.ae/uae/health/obesity-in-the-gulf-disturbing-new-survey#ixzz3LU
v6ZdR4.

24. Mourshed, Hediger, and Lambert, *Gulf Cooperation Council Health Care*, 56.

25. Ibid.

26. "QSA: Qatar's Population Has Nearly Doubled since 2007," *Doha News*, April 7, 2013,
http://dohanews.co/qsa-qatars-population-has-nearly-doubled-since-2007.

27. Mourshed, Hediger, and Lambert, *Gulf Cooperation Council Health Care*, 56.

28. Jawad A. Al-Lawati, Ruth Mabry, and Ali Jaffer Mohammed, "Addressing the Threat of
Chronic Diseases in Oman," *Preventing Chronic Disease* 5 (2008): 1, www.cdc.gov/pcd/issues
/2008/jul/pdf/07_0086.pdf.

29. Maria Kristiansen and Aziz Sheikh, "The Health of Low-Income Migrant Workers in
Gulf Cooperation Council Countries," *Health and Human Rights Journal*, July 22, 2014, www
.hhrjournal.org/2014/07/22/the-health-of-low-income-migrant-workers-in-gulf-cooperation
-council-countries/.

30. "UAE, Qatar Have Highest Expat Ratio in GCC," *Emirates 24/7*, September 11, 2013,
www.emirates247.com/news/emirates/uae-qatar-have-highest-expat-ratio-in-gcc-2013-09-11
-1.520659.

31. See "Medical Commission Procedures," Hukoomi Qatar e-Government Portal, http://
portal.www.gov.qa.

32. *The Economist*, "The New Unpeople: Statelessness as Punishment against Political
Dissent in the Gulf," November 15, 2014, www.economist.com/news/middle-east-and-africa
/21632640-statelessness-punishment-against-political-dissent-gulf-new-unpeople.

33. Michael C. Hudson, *Arab Politics: The Search for Legitimacy* (New Haven, CT: Yale
University Press, 1977), 85.

34. Shawn Teresa Flaniga and Mounah Abdel-Samad, "Hezbollah's Social Jihad: Nonprofits
as Resistance Organizations," *Middle East Policy* 16 (2009), www.mepc.org/journal/middle-east
-policy-archives/hezbollahs-social-jihad-nonprofits-resistance-organizations.

35. See, e.g., Viktor Hediger, Toby Lambert, and Mona Mourshed, "Private Solutions for
Health Care in the Gulf," *McKinsey Quarterly*, 2007.

36. Jennifer Bell, "Cleveland Clinic Abu Dhabi Opens Its Doors for First Patients," *The
National*, March 17, 2015, www.thenational.ae/uae/20150317/cleveland-clinic-abu-dhabi
-opens-its-doors-for-first-patients.

37. See *Strategic Alliances: The Role of Civil Society in Health*, Discussion Paper 1 (Geneva:
World Health Organization, 2001), www.who.int/civilsociety/documents/en/alliances_en.pdf.

38. This was highlighted by a Chatham House study group on Kuwait: "The extensive use
of foreign consultants has become particularly contentious because of the lack of local public

participation in economic debates. Participants were concerned that much of the knowledge about the Gulf is produced outside the region, partly because of local sensitivities to criticism and constraints on academic freedom." See Chatham House, "Kuwait Study Group: Citizenship and the Economy in the Gulf," May 24–25, 2013, 2, www.chathamhouse.org/sites/files /chathamhouse/field/field_document/20130524KuwaitStudyGroup.pdf.

39. Informa Exhibitions, "Healthcare in the GCC," 11.

40. Jay Loschky, "Snapshot: Many in GCC Prefer to Get Medical Treatment Abroad," Gallup, August 8, 2012, www.gallup.com/poll/156476/snapshot-gcc-prefer-medical-treatment -abroad.aspx.

41. "Life Evaluations in the GCC: Subjective Wellbeing and Health," Gallup, www.gallup .com/poll/157064/life-evaluations-gcc-subjective-wellbeing-health.aspx.

42. Mitya Underwood, "First-Rate Care on Your Doorstep When Cleveland Clinic Opens in Abu Dhabi," *The National*, October 13, 2014, www.thenational.ae/uae/health/first-rate-care-on -your-doorstep-when-cleveland-clinic-opens-in-abu-dhabi.

43. Latham & Watkins, "2013 Update: Healthcare Regulation in the United Arab Emirates," May 2003, www.lw.com/thoughtleadership/uae-healthcare-regulation-2013-update.

44. Alpen Capital, "GCC Healthcare Sector," April 22, 2014, 7, www.alpencapital.com /downloads/GCC_Healthcare_Sector_22_April_2014_Final.pdf.

45. "Kingdom of Saudi Arabia," BMJ Quality, http://quality.bmj.com/saudiarabia/.

46. "24% of QNRF Funding Goes to Healthcare and Medical Studies," *The Peninsula*, August 18, 2014, www.zawya.com/story/24_of_QNRF_funding_goes_to_healthcare_and _medical_studiesZAWYA2014081835924.

47. "Mapping the Qatari Genome to Prevent Inherited Diseases," Weill Cornell Medical College in Qatar, January 2014, http://qatar-weill.cornell.edu/media/reports/2013/qatari Genome.html.

48. Simeon Kerr, "Saudis Lead Healthcare Spending Spree," *Financial Times*, February 18, 2013, www.ft.com/intl/cms/s/0/8c82c150-79a4-11e2-9015-00144feabdc0.html#axzz3V6 NII4xO.

49. "WHO Definition of Health," World Health Organization, July 22, 1946, www.who .int/about/definition/en/print.html.

50. "Addressing the Burden of Cancer in the Gulf," *The Lancet*, December 2014, www.the lancet.com/pdfs/journals/lanonc/PIIS1470-2045(14)71141-6.pdf.

51. See, e.g., the country reports on Qatar and the United Arab Emirates in *World Report 2014*, Human Rights Watch, 2014, www.hrw.org/world-report/2014.

52. "Kuwait's Stateless Bidoon: Background and Recent Promising Developments," US Embassy in Kuwait, June 3, 2009, www.wikileaks.org/plusd/cables/09KUWAIT558_a.html.

53. Jane Kinninmont, "Citizenship in the Gulf," Chatham House, July 1, 2013, 52, www .chathamhouse.org/sites/files/chathamhouse/public/Research/Middle%20East/0713ch_kin ninmont.pdf.

54. *The Economist*, "The New Unpeople."

55. Thoraya Ahmed Obaid, "Islam, Globalization and Feminist Networks: Statement at the Annual Conference of the Middle East Studies Association (MESA) in Washington, DC," United Nations Population Fund, November 25, 2002, www.unfpa.org/news/statement -annual-conference-middle-east-studies-association-mesa-islam-globalization-and#sthash .o6uSjrCB.dpuf.

56. Farzaneh Roudi-Fahimi, "Gender and Equity in Access to Health Care Services in the Middle East and North Africa," Population Reference Bureau, 2006, www.prb.org/Publications

/Articles/2006/GenderandEquityinAccesstoHealthCareServicesintheMiddleEastandNorthAfrica
.aspx.

57. Ibid.

58. Mourshed, Hediger, and Lambert, *Gulf Cooperation Council Health Care*, 55.

59. Abdulwahab Alkhamis, Amir Hassan, and Peter Cosgrove, "Financing Healthcare in Gulf Cooperation Council Countries: A Focus on Saudi Arabia," *International Journal of Health Planning and Management* 29 (2014): 64–65.

60. Ibid., 78.

61. Naser Al Remeithi, "Many Emiratis Unaware of Thiqa's Mental Health Care Coverage," *The National*, March 5, 2015, www.thenational.ae/uae/many-emiratis-unaware-of-thiqas-mental-health-care-coverage.

62. Erik J. Koornneef, Paul B. M. Robben, Mohammed B. Al Seiari, and Zaid Al Siksek, "Health System Reform in the Emirate of Abu Dhabi, United Arab Emirates," *Health Policy* 108 (2012): 116.

63. Ibid., 116–17.

64. Ibid., 117.

65. Informa Exhibitions, "Healthcare in the GCC," 11.

66. Aspen Institute, *The Gulf Cooperation Council (GCC) and Health Worker Migration*, Global Policy Advisory Council Policy Brief, 1, www.aspeninstitute.org/sites/default/files/content/images/GCC%20and%20HWM%20Policy%20Brief.pdf.

67. Alpen Capital, "GCC Healthcare Sector," 53.

68. H. Hamdy, A. Telmesani, N. Al Wardy, et al., "Undergraduate Medical Education in the Gulf Cooperation Council: A Multi-Countries Study (Part 1)," *Medical Teacher* 32 (2010): 219.

69. Saudi Arabia's spending on healthcare falls within a broader budgetary category, that of "health and social affairs," which totals $29 billion; it is unclear what the exact amount directed toward healthcare solely is. See Alpen Capital, "GCC Healthcare Sector," 17; "Saudi Arabia's 2014 Budget Emphasizes Long-Term Development," US-Saudi Arabian Business Council, www.us-sabc.org/custom/news/details.cfm?id=1541.

70. Informa Exhibitions, "Healthcare in the GCC," 12.

71. See Supreme Council of Health, "Qatar National Health Accounts Report, 2011," June 2012, www.scribd.com/doc/101516164/Qatar-National-Health-Accounts-NHA-Report.

72. Supreme Council of Health, "Qatar Health Report 2012," April 2014, 50, www.nhsq.info/app/media/1479.

73. Ibid.

74. Bryant Ott, "GCC Residents Highly Satisfied with Healthcare Access," Gallup, March 8, 2012, www.gallup.com/poll/153155/gcc-residents-highly-satisfied-healthcare-access.aspx.

75. Supreme Council of Health, "Qatar Health Report 2012," 50.

76. "Strengthening Healthcare Systems in the GCC Countries Is Key to Improved Fairness and Accountability," World Bank, February 21, 2014, www.worldbank.org/en/news/press-release/2014/02/21/strengthening-healthcare-systems-in-the-gcc-countries.

77. Ibid.

HUMAN RESOURCES FOR HEALTHCARE IN THE GULF COOPERATION COUNCIL STATES

Mohamad Alameddine, Nour Kik, Rami Yassoub, and Yara Mourad

The Gulf Cooperation Council (GCC) region is characterized by rapid population growth backed up by strong economies and vibrant markets. However, despite considerable investments in healthcare infrastructure and re sources, the GCC states are still facing a plethora of challenges to provide the healthcare services that would ensure the health and well-being of their populations, both nationals and expatriates. Perhaps the most significant challenge for the effectiveness, efficiency, and sustainability of healthcare systems across the GCC is the continued availability of an adequate number of well-trained and experienced doctors, nurses, dentists, pharmacists, administrators, and other professionals who constitute human resources for health (HRH).

It is argued that the growth in HRH in the region, especially with regard to the workforce members who are nationals, neither matches the GCC's population growth nor satisfies its increasing needs. This has mandated the reliance on foreign trained, expatriate HRH. Yet, this excessive reliance on expatriate HRH has meant that the GCC states face the challenge of nationalizing the health workforce, an effort that is realizing varying degrees of success. Optimizing gender distribution and enhancing female participation in the healthcare workforce presents another challenge in the GCC states that is of pivotal importance, because it highly influences females' access to healthcare services, considering the religious, cultural, and social fabric of the society.

The overarching aim of this chapter is to investigate and critically scrutinize HRH trends in the GCC states in recent years. The chapter first offers concise country profiles that serve as a base for understanding local trends and specificities and reflects on the outcomes of past HRH reforms and initiatives. The chapter next turns to offering GCC comparisons with respect to HRH, in an attempt to decipher lessons learned and identify experiences and best practices that could be shared among the GCC states. Although the local specificities in the various GCC states are acknowledged, common themes and challenges are identified to guide a concerted regional effort in HRH management and planning.

The chapter is divided into four interrelated and complementary sections. The first section concisely highlights the importance of HRH and overviews the global and regional trends in HRH. The second offers six brief individual HRH country profiles outlining particular trends and challenges. The third provides overall GCC comparisons across key areas, including the ratio of HRH per population and the distribution of HRH by nationality (nationals vs. expatriates) and gender. And the fourth deciphers key lessons learned from past programs and initiatives to offer targeted recommendations that will assist the GCC states in strengthening the sustainability of their national capacities to attend to the capricious burden of disease that has recently expanded to include both the chronic and communicable maladies.

Although it is acknowledged that this chapter does not discuss profound country-specific programs for HRH development, it nevertheless attempts to concisely analyze key facts, figures, and past developments in order to offer evidence-informed recommendations for healthcare stakeholders and decision makers in the GCC member states on where things stand, and, more important, where future resources and efforts need to be focused.

AN OVERVIEW OF HUMAN RESOURCES FOR HEALTH

This section starts by highlighting the pivotal role played by HRH. It then offers a concise overview of global and regional HRH trends.

The Importance of Human Resources for Healthcare

HRH are the linchpin of any healthcare system. They include different types of healthcare providers across the biomedical team (physicians, nurses, etc.) as well as health management and support staff members (managers, accountants, engineers, etc.). Described as "the heart of the health system in any country," HRH are considered one of the key determinants of health services performance.[1] They are recognized by the World Health Organization's

Framework for Action for strengthening health systems as one of the six inter-related and interacting building blocks of health systems. Indeed, an adequate and well-distributed supply of skilled and motivated HRH working in a supportive environment is critical for health systems to respond to new challenges and provide effective health-improving services.[2] The number and qualifications of HRH are proven determinants of vital health indicators, including maternal mortality, infant mortality, and under-five-years mortality rates.[3] HRH also play an essential role in realizing universal health coverage.[4] With these factors in mind, strengthening the health workforce goes beyond enhancing organizational performance to ensuring that health systems can achieve national, regional, and global health goals.[5]

Considering the health implications of a steady supply of competent HRH, the *World Health Report 2006*, supported by recent global and regional efforts, stressed the urgency of addressing health workforce challenges, such as "shortages, imbalances, and mismatches between education models and health needs, and productivity concerns."[6]

Global Trends

When examining healthcare systems from a global perspective, general HRH issues related to the workforce's size, composition, distribution and training, migration of health workers, and cultural, economic, and sociodemographic factors stand out.[7] Healthcare systems face a striking and massive global shortage of health workers, including both healthcare providers and health management and support personnel.[8] This shortage is, in turn, expected to create an increasingly detrimental gap in health systems' infrastructure.[9]

Furthermore, health workers are severely maldistributed between regions and between states, a phenomenon exacerbated by unplanned international migration patterns that challenge countries' health system capacities.[10] Sub-Saharan Africa, for instance, has a tenth of the nurses and physicians for its population that Europe has.[11] In addition, the maldistribution of HRH between the public and private sectors is also evident in many countries.

The skewed gender distribution of HRH is also a global issue of concern. In many countries, females are concentrated in the lower-status healthcare occupations and represent a minority in the more highly trained professions (physicians, dentists, managers, etc.), resulting in a skewed distribution of females by professional category, in favor of nursing and midwifery personnel and other healthcare providers, such as community health workers.[12]

Focusing on HRH qualifications, skill imbalances are noted in almost all countries, causing widespread inefficiencies.[13] In some countries, the skill mix in healthcare is dominated by physicians and specialists, resulting in a neglected workforce for population-based public health.[14]

In light of the suboptimal planning that yielded the misdistributions described above, HRH issues have grown into major global health policy concerns.[15] In the Eastern Mediterranean Region (EMR) countries, in particular, weaknesses in HRH development planning constitute one of the most crucial issues facing healthcare systems, with problems ranging from an absolute shortage to underemployment and skills imbalances, in addition to geographical maldistribution.[16] These setbacks have provided the EMR with the second-lowest number of HRH after Africa, and have contributed to an overwhelming three-quarters of HRH being health/biomedical service providers.[17] Further examination of regional flows of providers reveals that lower-income Arab countries are generally "donors" of nurses and physicians, whereas higher-income GCC states are "recipients."[18]

Regional Trends

The GCC aims at enhancing coordination, integration, and interconnections between its member states in all fields in order to support individual states' efforts through the unity provided by the council.[19] The GCC member states are high-income Arab Islamic countries characterized by abundant natural resources and a high gross domestic product. In 2011, the GCC states' gross domestic product per capita was $30,000, whereas the global average was about $10,000.[20]

Furthermore, the GCC states are characterized by population growth rates that are among the highest in the world, reaching a total population close to 46 million individuals in 2011 (table 3.1). The total GCC population is projected to reach 53.41 million in 2020.[21] Continued high population growth will create shortages not only of health resources but also of energy and water. Unsurprisingly, the GCC states are also characterized by a high or very high human development index.[22]

With a predominant reliance on expatriates to meet local healthcare demands, evident from the fact that foreign workers constituted the majority of physicians in all the GCC's states in 2006, the GCC was unable to supply enough clinical staff to meet acceptable ratios of providers to population.[23] For this and other policy and sustainability matters of concern, all the GCC states

Table 3.1   **Populations of the GCC States, 2008–11**

Country	2008	2009	2010	2011	% increase, 2008–11
Saudi Arabia	25,787,025	26,660,857	27,136,977	28,376,355	10.04
United Arab Emirates	8,073,626	8,199,996	8,264,070	8,925,100[a]	10.55
Oman	2,867,000	3,173,917	2,773,000	3,295,298	14.94
Kuwait	2,495,851	2,583,020	2,672,926	3,065,850	22.84
Qatar	1,448,479	1,638,644	1,699,435	1,732,717	19.62
Bahrain	1,106,509	1,178,415	1,228,543	1,195,020	8.00
Total	41,778,490	43,434,849	43,774,951	45,929,310	9.94

Sources: Information Sector, Statistical Department for the GCC Secretariat General, "Statistical Bulletin," 2012, http://sites.gcc-sg.org/DLibrary/download.php?B=633; World Bank, "Country Demographic Profiles," 2014, http://data.worldbank.org/country.

[a] The United Arab Emirates' 2011 population numbers were retrieved from World Bank, "Country Demographic Profiles: United Arab Emirates," http://databank.worldbank.org/data/views/reports/tableview.aspx.

have been engaging in strong and explicit labor nationalization efforts.[24] Most of their policies, however, have faced implementation problems because only minimal research and knowledge—which are imperative for proper policy planning, policymaking, and program evaluation—have been developed to inform and direct decision makers.[25]

A representative example is the initiative to strengthen existing medical education efforts through the GCC members' collaborations with European and US medical schools. The fact is that, despite these efforts, it was predicted that not enough medical graduates would be generated to keep pace with the GCC's population increase and, thus, its reliance on foreign-trained physicians and nurses is expected to continue for the foreseeable future.[26]

Overall, the GCC's demand for healthcare is anticipated to increase by 240 percent in the next twenty years, the highest among all regions in the world.[27] It is therefore unmistakably imperative to strengthen the health workforce to counter the effects of crippling diseases and their associated economic burdens. Closing the HRH supply/demand gap is essential to address current and future anticipated needs of the GCC's population, both nationals and expatriates.[28] However, in order to better decide on modes for alleviating the HRH undersupply and unearth the main challenges facing the region's health systems, a thorough assessment of the GCC's recent and ongoing HRH workforce quantities and developments is needed. Such an assessment will be essential for guiding the planning and management of HRH.[29]

APPROACHES

To conduct this thorough assessment of the GCC's HRH workforce, we systematically explored the published literature and statistical reports of all GCC member states. First, the ministries' or other health authorities' websites for each GCC country were examined, and the national HRH databases were analyzed when available. Second, regional and international organizations' websites, in addition to both peer-reviewed publications and white and gray papers, were reviewed for HRH indicators and figures.

The keywords used in our search were human resources for health; HRH ratios/proportions/distribution; healthcare system; health manpower; health workforce; health professionals; physicians; nurses; pharmacists; allied health professionals (AHP); healthcare sectors; HRH development; HRH development programs, HRH training; HRH recruitment/retention; HRH planning capacity; GCC; Saudi Arabia; Bahrain; Kuwait; Qatar; the United Arab Emirates; and Oman. The regions and countries that were included in the search were the following:

Regions: EMR; Middle East, Arab countries; GCC
Countries: Bahrain, Oman, Kuwait, Qatar, the United Arab Emirates, and Saudi Arabia

Univariate descriptive analyses were generated. Trends were analyzed by professional category, nationality, gender, and sector of employment (public vs. private) when the relevant data were available. Staffing ratios of HRH by population were also analyzed and compared.

The objective of this review was not to compile an exhaustive list of articles and reports but rather to formulate an overview of HRH trends, issues, and opportunities in the GCC region by integrating scattered data for convenient modeling and analytical purposes. Taking into consideration that published numbers and estimates might differ between references, the figures published by the Ministry of Health (MOH) and health authorities were the ones deemed valid and reliable and were used to draw country profiles and comparisons. To better guide the reader, the source of numbers utilized in each of the sections is clearly highlighted. Whenever possible, the numbers and trends provided were triangulated with other literature sources in order to cross-validate them and ensure the deciphering of accurate policy and practice recommendations. Due to the unavailability of data analyses at the country and GCC levels, we focus here on these professions: physicians, nurses, pharmacists, and dentists. Other AHPs were included in comparisons whenever data were available.

HUMAN RESOURCES FOR HEALTH IN THE GULF COOPERATION COUNCIL STATES

This section offers brief HRH profiles for each GCC state, outlining key trends and challenges. Although some of the reported trends and challenges are unique to the country context, others are crosscutting among a number of GCC states.

Saudi Arabia

In 2012 the total health manpower working in Saudi Arabia was distributed as follows: 71,518 physicians, 10,002 dentists, 139,701 nurses, 15,590 pharmacists, and 76,769 AHPs.[30] As such, in 2012, there were 2.3 nurses for every physician employed in Saudi Arabia, in comparison with 1.3 nurses for every physician in the EMR and 1.8 nurses for every physician globally, according to the World Health Organization's *World Health Statistics Report 2013.*[31]

As exhibited in figure 3.1, the period between 2008 and 2012 witnessed a steady growth in the number of HRH in Saudi Arabia across all professional groups (with the exception of pharmacists). This growth was most pronounced

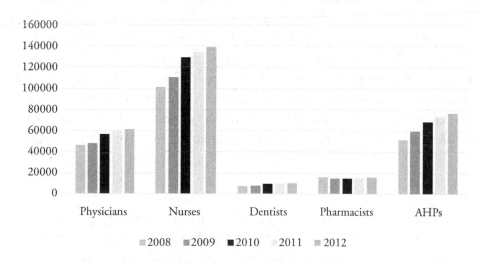

Figure 3.1   **Health Professionals in Saudi Arabia, 2008–12**

Source: Economist Intelligence Unit, "The GCC in 2020: The Gulf and Its People," 2009, http://graphics.eiu.com/upload/eb/Gulf2020part2.pdf.

for AHPs (48.9 percent). Significant increases were also noted in numbers of dentists (44.1 percent), nurses (37.9 percent), and physicians (32.4 percent). Despite the observed increase in the number of health professionals, future needs are likely to result in shortages in part because of the anticipated increased average age of the populations within each GCC state.

The proportion of Saudis among the health workforce has steadily increased between 2008 and 2012 as well as across all professional categories.[32] Nevertheless, as of 2012, the proportion of Saudis among health workers remains low in all categories except AHPs: physicians (23.8 percent), nurses (36.2 percent), pharmacists (19.4 percent), and AHPs (72.0 percent).[33] On that front, the Saudi Board for Medical Specialization had estimated that by 2020, Saudi Arabia will still be in need of 32,660 physicians and 52,420 nurses from other countries.[34] Correcting the existing imbalances will require advanced planning and a substantial resource investment.

During the period 2008–12, the change in the proportion of Saudi HRH differed significantly between the public and private healthcare sectors. The overall change within the public sector was about 72 percent, whereas that in the private sector was only 21 percent. For the public sector, the professional group that witnessed the highest increase in its Saudi workforce was the AHPs (77.1 percent), followed by nurses (73.9 percent). For the private sector, the highest increase was observed for physicians (64.5 percent), with pharmacists and nurses witnessing a drop in their Saudi workforce (–44.8 percent and –7.0 percent, respectively; see figure 3.2).

For 2012, the proportion of females within the healthcare workforce was as follows: physicians, including dentists (27.8 percent); nurses (79.6 percent); pharmacists (38.8 percent); and AHPs (31.3 percent). Training or recruiting female physicians to narrow this gender gap remains a challenge for all the GCC states. The overall proportion of female HRH was 53.6 percent. The large number of female nurses leads to a more equitable gender ratio in the overall HRH data.

Bahrain

Bahrain also witnessed varying developments in its HRH availability, depending on the HRH profession. As seen in figure 3.3, the ratios of physicians and nurses and midwives per 10,000 persons grew significantly during the period 2008–12. The growth rate seems particularly striking between 2010 and 2012. These increases were paralleled by a growth in the ratio of beds per 10,000 persons between 2010 and 2011. As a result, the country has the second-highest physi-

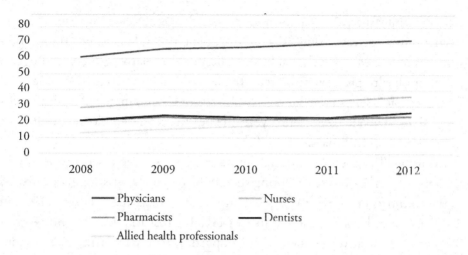

Figure 3.2 **Distribution of Human Resources for Health in Saudi Arabia by Professional Category, 2008–12 (per 10,000 population)**

Source: Saudi Arabian Ministry of Health, "Health Statistics Book for the Year 1433," 2012, http://www.moh.gov.sa/en/ministry/statistics/book/documents/1433.pdf.

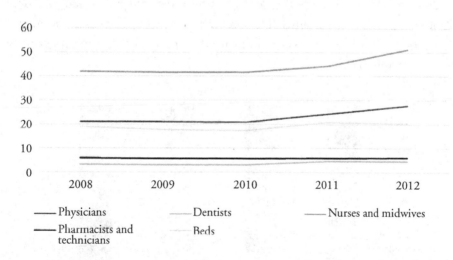

Figure 3.3 **Distribution of Human Resources for Health in Bahrain by Professional Category, 2008–12 (per 10,000 population)**

Source: Alpen Capital, "GCC Healthcare Industry," 2014, http://www.alpencapital.com /downloads/GCC_Healthcare_Sector_22_April_2014_Final.pdf.

cian availability per 10,000 persons in the GCC region, following Qatar.[35] Apart from a minor increase from 2010 to 2011, the ratio of dentists per 10,000 persons has remained relatively stable. Also, despite the relative growth in the rates of certain health professions, as reported by Bahrain's Economic Development Board, employment in the Bahraini health sector has not matched the industry's expansion, of about 10 percent a year; the health sector's employment rate had grown by about half that as of 2009.[36]

Additionally, though the overall number of nurses increased noticeably in Bahrain's government sector during the 2008–12 period, it strongly decreased in the country's private sector. These sharp changes occurred between 2010 and 2011. Overall, however, the number of HRH across the different professions has remained relatively stable.[37] The proportion of HRH in the government sector increased by 52.1 percent between 2008 and 2012, whereas that in the private sector decreased by 51.9 percent.

With regard to the proportion of nationals to expatriates, Bahraini HRH outnumber non-Bahrainis in the majority of health professions, as illustrated in figure 3.4. In particular, the overwhelming majority of pharmacists (98 percent) and dentists (94 percent) are Bahrainis. Furthermore, more than half of nurses (52 percent) are non-Bahrainis. The encouraging proportions may be further enhanced with the recent drives to improve the uptake of training programs by Bahraini nationals.[38]

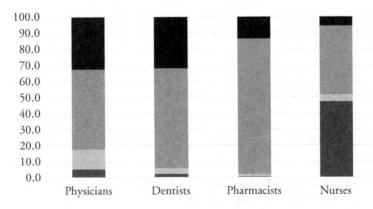

■ Non-Bahraini females ▨ Non-Bahraini males ■ Bahraini females ■ Bahraini males

Figure 3.4 **Distribution of Human Resources for Health in Bahrain by Professional Category, Nationality, and Gender, 2012**

Source: Oxford Business Group, "Bahrain Continues to See Rapid Growth in the Healthcare Sector," April 15, 2014, http://www.oxfordbusinessgroup.com/news/bahrain -continues-see-rapid-growth-health-care-sector.

A striking observation noted within the HRH distribution by professional category and gender in 2012 is the domination of females in all four categories, as seen in figure 3.5. Females constituted an overwhelming 90.4 percent of nurses, 84.7 percent of pharmacists, 64.8 percent of dentists, and 55.2 percent of physicians, with the highest representation of females being among non-Bahraini female nurses. Thus, in this country female health professionals are available to female patients if they prefer being cared for by a female.

Qatar

According to the former Qatar Statistics Authority, there was an increase in the ratio of physicians per 10,000 persons from 21 in 1998 to 33 in 2009, a density comparable to that for developed countries.[39] The ratio of nurses per 10,000 persons also increased during this period, reaching 62 in 2010.[40]

Despite a decrease between 2008 and 2009 in all categories except physicians, as seen in figure 3.6, a sharp increase in HRH followed between 2009 and 2010. In addition to the growing number of healthcare professionals, numerous new internationally recognized institutions have launched their initiatives in Qatar, thus considerably improving the quality of the healthcare delivery in the country.[41]

In 2012 Qatar had 10,649 nurses (making up 47.4 percent of the total health workforce), 4,637 physicians (20.6 percent), 1,787 pharmacists and pharmacist

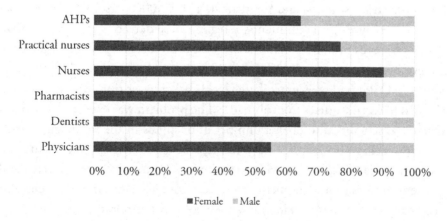

Figure 3.5 **Distribution of Human Resources for Health in Bahrain by Professional Category and Gender, 2012**

Source: Data from Ministry of Health–Health Information Directorate, Bahrain, "Health Statistics 2012."

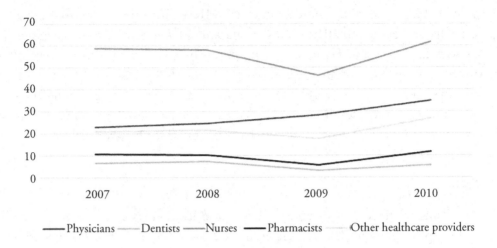

Figure 3.6   **Distribution of Human Resources for Health in Qatar by Professional Category, 2007–10 (per 10,000 population)**

Source: Abdulbari Bener and Ahmed Al Mazroei, "Health Services Management in Qatar," *Croatian Medical Journal* 51, no. 1 (2010): 85–88.

assistants (8.0 percent), and 1,152 dentists (5.1 percent).[42] Other medical and AHPs (including laboratory technicians, radiographers, and physiotherapists) constituted about 19.0 percent of the total health workforce.

The health workforce density in 2012 was 58.1 nurses, 25.3 physicians, 6.3 pharmacists and assistants, and 9.7 dentists per 10,000 persons.[43] Perhaps because of more vigorous recruitment strategies, these densities were higher than the GCC averages but lower than the Organization for Economic Cooperation and Development averages.[44] Officials had said that the long-standing shortage of nurses in Qatar had been exacerbated by global competition, which was making it hard to recruit nurses from abroad.[45] The problem was expected to worsen as Qatar was scheduled to open a number of hospitals in the following years.[46] These large demands on HRH have resulted in an overwhelming reliance on a health expatriate workforce, with an estimated 69 percent of physicians and 91 percent of nurses in Qatar being recruited from abroad. Of greater concern is that many of these expatriates view their jobs as temporary.[47] Furthermore, members of the expatriate healthcare workforce may require additional language training or special training relating to cultural awareness.

Data on the distribution of Qatar's health workforce by nationality and gender are supported by statistics from the Supreme Council of Health (SCH) and Hamad Medical Corporation (HMC). It is worth noting here that the workforce in SCH and HMC is quite representative of the country's health workforce as a whole because HMC alone provides more than 90 percent of the curative services, and, hence, is a large employer of HRH in the country, and because, as mentioned above, the public sector (along with the Primary Healthcare Corporation—the primary public healthcare provider) is the largest employer of HRH in Qatar.[48] In 2012 all professional categories among the medical staff members working at SCH and HMC were overwhelmingly dominated by non Qataris. In total, only 8.21 percent of the total health workforce in SCH and HMC were Qatari—but, encouragingly enough, 79.8 percent were females. In fact, females constituted the majority of the Qatari health workforce at SCH and HMC across all health categories (fig. 3.7). Notably, Qatari males constituted a very small proportion of the health workforce across all categories, making up only 5.9 percent of physicians, 0.01 percent of nurses, 0.5 percent of pharmacists and assistant pharmacists, and 1.5 percent of other medical staff members and AHPs. With regard to nurses, in 2012 there was only 1 Qatari male nurse (0.01 percent) and 241 Qatari female nurses (3 percent), versus 1,095 non-Qatari male nurses (13.6 percent) and 6,697 non-Qatari female nurses (83.4 percent). As such, one of the main challenges that Qatar still

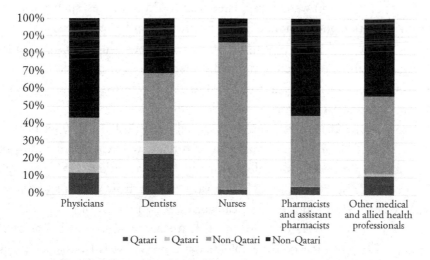

Figure 3.7 **Medical Staff Working at the Supreme Council of Health and Hamad Medical Corporation, by Nationality and Gender, 2012**

Source: Hamad Medical Corporation, "Annual Health Report 2012," 2013, http://site .hmc.org.qa/msrc/ahr.htm.

faces is its dependence on foreign medical professionals.[49] Recruitment and re-tention of the appropriate healthcare workforce members have indeed become increasingly difficult in Qatar.[50] To address some of these manpower issues, a new medical school has recently opened in Doha that is aimed at recruiting and retaining medical students from Qatar.

In terms of the public–private mix, although the numbers of HRH in Qatar have grown considerably over a relatively short period (2007–10) in both the private and the governmental sectors, the increase has been much more pronounced in the private sector (91.6 percent vs. 50.0 percent in the governmental sector between 2007 and 2010).[51] Nevertheless, the governmental sector still employed 66.6 percent of the total health workforce in 2012.[52]

Requiring special consideration is the distribution of HRH within the same health category. The numbers of general practitioners and specialists both witnessed a strong increase between 2005 and 2012; however, the overall increase in the number of specialists (128.2 percent) was much higher than that of general practitioners (75.7 percent).[53] For many physicians, specialization rather than a general practice appears to be a more attractive career option.

Kuwait

HRH data for Kuwait were extrapolated from various sources, such as the World Health Statistics, the Regional Office for the Eastern Mediterranean, and the Regional Bureau of Health Ministers of the GCC, in addition to some country-specific indicators.[54] As seen in figure 3.8, the number of physicians and nurses per 10,000 persons increased from 2003 to 2012, whereas the numbers of dentists and pharmacists remained relatively stable.

According to 2012 data from the Central Statistical Bureau, 84 percent of Kuwait's health workforce is made up of foreign workers.[55] Both the private and public health sectors were dominated by foreign workers (95.6 percent and 80.4 percent, respectively, in 2012), mostly coming from South and Southeast Asia.[56] Classified into professional categories, 94.1 percent of nurses, 66.3 percent of physicians, and 48.5 percent of dentists were non-Kuwaiti as of 2012 (fig. 3.9). Despite their considerable demand, very few Kuwaitis are engaging in a nursing career,[57] with the proportion of Kuwaitis among nurses working in the MOH only mildly increasing, from 7.4 percent in 2008 to 7.5 percent in 2012.[58] Furthermore, the proportion of Kuwaiti physicians decreased from 40.7 percent in 2008 to 39.8 percent in 2012. However, it is forecasted that this proportion is going to increase to 51.9 percent of the national need by 2020.[59]

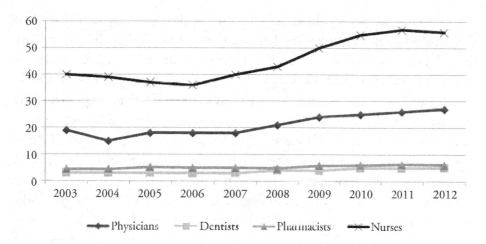

Figure 3.8 **Distribution of Human Resources for Health in Kuwait by Professional Category, 2003–12 (per 10,000 population)**

Source: Data from Kuwait Central Statistical Bureau, "Annual Bulletin of the Health Statistics 2012," 2013, www.csb.gov.kw/Socan_Statistic_EN.aspx?ID=59.

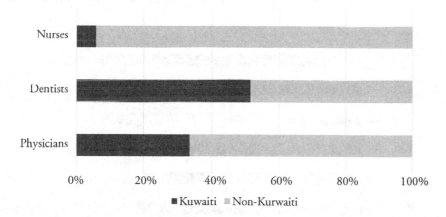

Figure 3.9 **Distribution of Nurses, Dentists, and Physicians in Kuwait by Nationality, 2012**

Source: Kuwait Central Statistical Bureau, "Annual Bulletin of the Health Statistics 2012," 2013, http://www.csb.gov.kw/Socan_Statistic_EN.aspx?ID=59; Ben Garcia, "Few Arabs Take Up Nursing as a Career," *Kuwait Times*, March 22, 2014, http://news.kuwaittimes .net/arabs-take-nursing-career/.

Examining the gender distribution of the medical workforce, it is evident that feminization has undergone key transformations during the past twenty years.[60] The ratio of males to females decreased from 2.2:1 in 2005 to 1:1 in 2010. This was expected because during the past decade, the number of female medical graduates has increased from 10 percent to more than 50 percent. The increase in female medical graduates is supported by medical schools' acceptance and admission rates.[61] Nevertheless, female physicians are more likely to choose nonsurgical specialties, work fewer hours in patient care settings, and generally retire earlier than their male counterparts.[62]

All the more, in 2012, females constituted 62 percent of the total health workforce in Kuwait. This can be explained, as seen in figure 3.10, by the fact that the nurses category—which, by far, is the largest in the country—is dominated by females (78.6 percent). Otherwise, males dominate all other professional categories except that of medical technicians. Physicians were the category with the highest proportion of males (64.8 percent), followed by dentists (62.4 percent).

With regard to the public–private mix, the private sector employs the lowest number of HRH per 10,000 persons, and the majority of those employed are nurses, who in 2011 amounted to only 8 per 10,000 persons, compared with

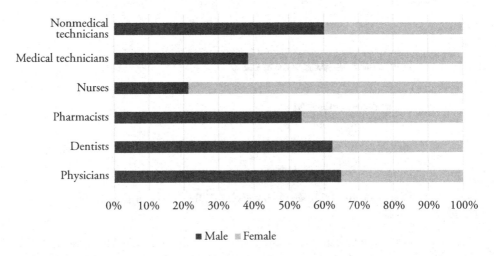

Figure 3.10 **Distribution of Human Resources for Health in Kuwait by Professional Category and Gender, 2012**

Sources: Peter Brooks, Helen M. Lapsley, and David Butt, "Medical Workforce Issues in Australia: 'Tomorrow's Doctors-Too Few, Too Far,'" *Medical Journal of Australia* 179, no. 4 (2003): 206; US Department of Health and Human Services, "Physician Supply and Demand: Projections to 2020," 2006, http://bhpr.hrsa.gov/healthworkforce /supplydemand/medicine/physician2020projections.pdf.

52 per 10,000 persons in the national sector and 44 per 10,000 persons in the MOH alone. The number of physicians in 2010 and 2011 was comparable in both the MOH and the national sector: 17 and 19 per 10,000 persons, respectively, as per 2011 data. The same applies to dentists for the same year: 3.5 and 3.7 per 10,000, respectively. The overall availability of HRH increased by about 10 percent across all categories and in all sectors between 2010 and 2011 (except for the dentist category in the private sector).

At the level of health facilities and equipment, the growth in beds per 10,000 persons between 2006 and 2012 was closely paralleled by the growth in the number of hospital nurses per bed. Indeed, the number of hospital nurses per bed increased by 26.3 percent between 2003 and 2012. The number of hospital physicians per bed also increased, by 22.2 percent.

With major expansions in Kuwait's hospital infrastructure, the demand for medical personnel is expected to rise. It is noted that 4,000 physicians and 10,000 nurses were needed to staff new hospitals by 2016.[63]

The United Arab Emirates

In 2012 the United Arab Emirates was facing a worrying shortfall of physicians, with a low ratio of physicians per 10,000 persons compared with developed countries like the United States and some European countries.[64] As such, an urgent recruitment drive to hire thousands of new physicians was launched.[65] Abu Dhabi alone planned to increase the number of physicians by more than 40 percent over a five-year period because it needed an additional 3,100 physicians by 2020, according to the Health Authority of Abu Dhabi (HAAD).[66] The need for additional physicians, among other HRH, was highlighted by HAAD statistics, which revealed that there were only 16 physicians per 10,000 persons in Abu Dhabi, with specific and severe shortages in cardiology and in neonatal, emergency, and critical and intensive care. HAAD was planning to increase this ratio to 23 per 10,000 persons during the next five years, with Emiratis constituting at least a quarter of the total workforce increase.[67]

During 2013, other nongovernmental sources have put the number of physicians and nurses in the United Arab Emirates at 15 and 27 per 10,000 persons, respectively, lower than in Qatar, Oman, and Kuwait.[68] As such, despite the consistent growth in the numbers of physicians, nurses, and beds over the past decade, the United Arab Emirates is lagging behind both developed markets across the world and neighboring markets in the GCC. The need for additional physicians to meet the healthcare requirements of the increasing population in the United Arab Emirates is significant, with the compound annual growth rate in the number of physicians over the next decade estimated to range from 3.4 percent to 9 percent. Internal medicine, general radiology, surgery, and anesthesiology are likely to witness key growth trajectories.[69] As seen in figure 3.11, only 7.9 percent of nurses, 19.2 percent of physicians, and 32.3 percent of technicians employed by the MOH are Emirati. Even though 86.2 percent of nontechnicians, 63.9 percent of pharmacists, and 58.7 percent of dentists are Emirati, overall, Emiratis constitute only 33.2 percent of the health work-force employed by the MOH. According to data from HAAD, nationals of the United Arab Emirates only constituted 10 percent of all physicians in the Abu Dhabi Emirate in 2012, a number that can partly be explained by the chal-lenges in attracting and retaining quality staff.[70] This low level of nationaliza-tion is especially problematic because it is quite common for nurses and AHPs to use their experience in the United Arab Emirates as a launchpad to practice medicine in bigger and more established markets, typically spending only three to five years in the country. This pattern is significantly burdening concerned healthcare organizations.[71]

The need for Emiratis in the healthcare professions, therefore, is pressing. As such, health leaders are advocating for better postgraduate medical education to

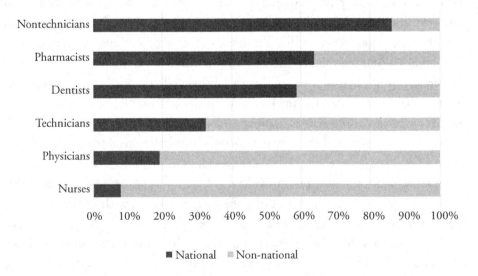

Figure 3.11   **Distribution of Human Resources for Health in the Ministry of Health of the United Arab Emirates, by Professional Category and Nationality, 2012**

Source: Data from Ministry of Health, United Arab Emirates, 2012, www.moh.gov.ae /en/OpenData/Pages/OpenData.aspx?Category=Statistics; manpower by category, medical district, nationality, and sex.

motivate domestic talent, and for more physicians to be trained locally to reduce the high turnover of expatriate employees.[72]

Despite the shortcomings in HRH availability at the level of density per population, the quantity of HRH has been increasing in the United Arab Emirates in absolute numbers; although it has been an uneven distribution between the public and private sectors. According to further data from the United Arab Emirates' National Bureau of Statistics, the numbers of physicians, dentists, and nurses in the emirates' government sector remained relatively steady during the period 2007–12, with only a slight increase in the number of nurses. In contrast, the United Arab Emirates' private sector witnessed substantial increases in the numbers of HRH during that same period, with physicians and dentists nearly doubling and nurses quadrupling in number. As such, in 2012, 84.5 percent of dentists, 68 percent of physicians, and 50.8 percent of nurses were employed in the private sector (figs. 3.12 and 3.13).

Oman

In Oman, interest in human resources development has been a priority for the past few decades and has been looked on as a strategy for achieving effective health services development. Accordingly, HRH availability in the sultanate has grown significantly over the years.[73] Oman has also been keen on achieving total

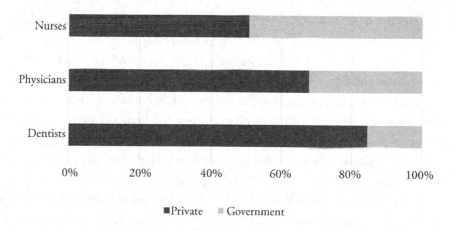

Figure 3.12   **Distribution of Human Resources in Health in the United Arab Emirates by Professional Category and Sector, 2012**

Source: Data from Ministry of Health, United Arab Emirates, 2012, www.moh.gov.ae /en/OpenData/Pages/OpenData.aspx?Category=Statistics; manpower by category, medical district, nationality, and sex.

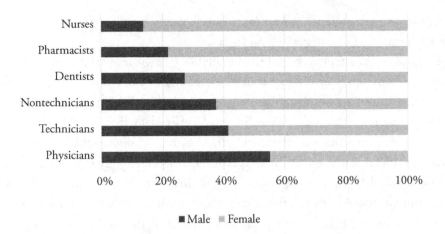

Figure 3.13 **Distribution of Human Resources in Health in the United Arab Emirates by Professional Category and Gender, 2012**

Source: Data from Ministry of Health, United Arab Emirates, 2012, www.moh.gov.ae /en/OpenData/Pages/OpenData.aspx?Category=Statistics; manpower by category, medical district, nationality, and sex.

self-reliance in terms of supply of physicians and has thus been pursuing policies and plans over the past years for that purpose.[74]

Increases in HRH numbers are clearly observed in figure 3.14. Between 1990 and 2012, the ratio of HRH per 10,000 persons across all categories increased significantly. The most considerable increases were in the numbers of nurses and physicians. These increases yielded the following HRH density rates, as per 2012 accounts: for every 10,000 persons, there were 19.5 physicians and 43.1 nurses in the country, as compared with 9.0 physicians and 26.0 nurses in 1990.

According to the statistics of the Omani MOH, the HRH increases given above may be one cause of the number of hospital beds per physician strongly and steadily decreasing during the period from 1990 to 2012, from 2.5 to 1.0 beds per physician. Likewise, the number of hospital beds per nurse also considerably decreased, from 1.4 to 0.4 beds per nurse.

The Omanization rate in the MOH during the period 1990–2012 increased in all medical and paramedical categories. The increase among physicians was from 9 percent in 1990 to 36 percent in 2012, while among nurses there was an increase from 12 percent in 1990 to 66 percent in 2012. Examining the Omanization rate in the total health workforce in the sultanate in 2012, as seen in figure 3.15, the highest proportions of Omanis were in the AHPs category. Only 29 percent of physicians and 27 percent of pharmacists were Omani. A higher proportion of Omanis was reported in the nurses category (54 percent).

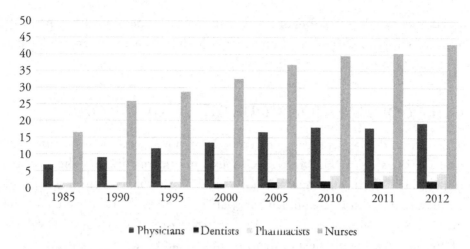

Figure 3.14 **Distribution of Human Resources in Health in Oman by Professional Category, 1985–2012 (per 10,000 population)**

Source: Data from Ministry of Health, Sultanate of Oman, *Annual Health Report*, 2012, www.moh.gov.om/en/stat/2012/index_eng.htm.

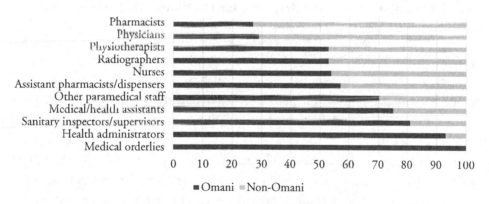

Figure 3.15 **Distribution of Human Resources in Health in Oman by Professional Category and Nationality, 2012**

Source: Data from Ministry of Health, Sultanate of Oman, *Annual Health Report*, 2012, www.moh.gov.om/en/stat/2012/index_eng.htm.

With regard to the gender distribution of HRH employed in the MOH of Oman, females dominated the categories of nurses (88.4 percent), pharmacists (70.6 percent), medical orderlies (67.0 percent), laboratory technicians (60.0 percent), assistant pharmacists (54.3 percent), and other paramedical staff (52.7 percent). Overall, females constituted 63.8 percent of Oman's health workforce. However, this could have been due to the overwhelming number of nurses within the MOH workforce as compared with other categories. Indeed, males still dominated the categories of sanitary inspectors / supervisors (95.8 percent), administrators (89.6 percent), physicians (58.6 percent), dentists (57.2 percent), and radiographers (55.4 percent).

GULF COOPERATION COUNCIL COMPARISONS

This section displays comparisons across the six GCC states in availability and characteristics of HRH. More specifically, the section displays the distribution of HRH by professional category, gender, nationality (national vs. nonnational), and sector of employment (public vs. private), all of which are key health systems indicators of vital importance to the GCC states. The focus of comparisons for physicians, dentists, nurses, and pharmacists is due to the limited availability of data for other health professionals. We have utilized the most recent available data and have compared country figures for similar years, unless otherwise indicated.

The Distribution of Human Resources for Health by Professional Category

In all six GCC states, the majority of HRH are distributed in the health service providers' categories of nurses and midwives, physicians, pharmaceutical personnel, and dentistry personnel. Although Bahrain had the highest proportion of physicians per population in 2012, Qatar had the highest proportions of nurses, pharmacists, and dentists per population compared with the other GCC states (fig. 3.16).

In 2012, the ratio of nurses to physicians in all GCC states was either equal to or exceeded that of the regional (1.3 nurses per physician) and global averages (1.8 nurses per physician). It ranged from a low of 1.8 nurses per physician in Bahrain to a high of 2.4 nurses per physician in Qatar, Kuwait, and Saudi Arabia.

Shortages of Physicians and Medical Staff

Significant shortages of local and skilled staff members are noticeable in all the GCC states, with a dominance of expatriates in both the nursing and physician fields. Despite nationalization efforts, the availability of medical personnel in several countries is not in line with their growing populations.[75] The medical industry in the GCC is indeed struggling to find suitable talent, mainly because the region is not producing enough medical graduates to meet the needs of the growing population.[76]

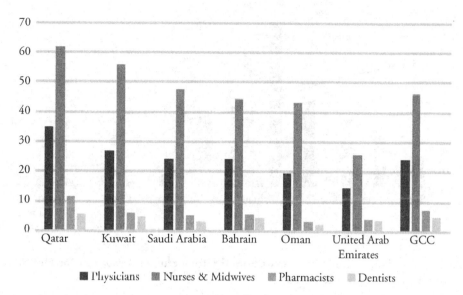

Figure 3.16   **Distribution of Human Resources for Health in the GCC Countries by Professional Category, 2012 (per 10,000 population)**

Source: Data from World Health Organization, "Regional Health Observatory Data Repository," 2013, http://rho.emro.who.int/rhodata/?theme=country

Note: For Bahrain and Saudi Arabia, nurses include midwives. For Qatar, pharmacists include assistants.

In the region, healthcare indicators such as bed density, physician density, and nurse density currently lag behind those of developed economies.[77] More specifically, for physicians, the shortage is further challenged by needs for higher standards of medical practice.[78] As such, health institutions are driven to recruit most of their clinical staff members from foreign countries.[79]

The Distribution of Human Resources for Health by Nationality

The vast majority of the GCC's HRH is foreign born and trained, with an estimated 75 percent of the physicians and 79 percent of the nurses working in the GCC states in 2008 being expatriates trained in more than fifty different countries.[80] This multiplicity in academic professional backgrounds has resulted in inconsistencies in techniques and training standards across the region, as a recent study has found.[81] Having said this, it is noteworthy that the nationalization strategies of HRH have had varying degrees of success by country and across diverse professions.

Figure 3.17 reveals that Bahrain indeed stands out in the nationalization of its physician, dentist, and pharmacist workforces but lags behind Oman in the

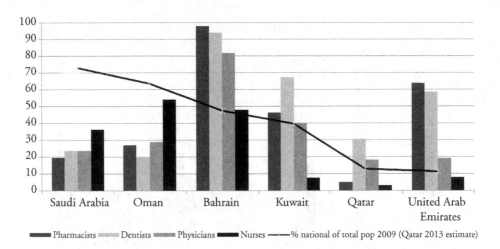

Figure 3.17   **Proportion of Nationals from the Total Human Resources for Health across the GCC Countries, 2012**

Sources: Kingdom of Saudi Arabia, Ministry of Health, "Annual Health Statistics Report 2012," 2013; Sultanate of Oman, Ministry of Health, "Oman Annual Health Report 2012," 2012, http://ghdx.healthdata.org/record/oman-annual-health-report-2012; Bahrain Ministry of Health, "MOH HRH Statistics Report 2012," 2013; United Arab Emirates, Ministry of Health, "MOH Manpower Statistics 2012," 2012; Kuwait Central Statistical Bureau, "Annual Bulletin of Health Statistics 2012," 2013, http://www.csb.gov.kw/Socan_Statistic_EN.aspx?ID=59; Hamad Medical Corporation, "Annual Health Report 2012"; Cooperation Council for the Arab States of the Gulf, "Gulf Cooperation Council: A Statistical Glance," 2012, http://sites.gcc-sg.org/DLibrary/index-eng.php?action=ShowBooks&SID=2.

Note: Proportions are reported from the MOH HRH for Kuwait and the United Arab Emirates and from the Hamad Medical Corporation and Supreme Council of Health in Qatar.

nationalization of its nursing workforce. On this front, Oman leads the other Gulf states, because it is the only country in the region whose proportion of nurses who are nationals exceeds that of those who are expatriates. In contrast, fewer than one in ten nurses working in Qatar, the United Arab Emirates, and Kuwait are nationals. Comparing health professionals, the physician and nursing workforces appear to be in need of the most attention because the majority of the workforce in all the GCC states, except for physicians in Bahrain and nurses in Oman, are nonnationals.

It could be argued that the large proportion of expatriate HRH may care for the equally high proportion of nonnational residents in GCC states. To make a more meaningful comparison and examine this argument, figure 3.17 portrays a line that exhibits the proportion of expatriates out of the total population in each of the GCC states. These proportions provided for all GCC states are for

2009, except for Qatar, where the proportion for 2012 was calculated based on the triangulation of a number of sources because it was not available from official sources.[82] A proportion of HRH personnel who are nationals below the line means that such a proportion would be insufficient to care for the population of nationals. Based on this, two facts become quite evident. First, all the GCC states, except for Bahrain, suffer from a severe shortage of locally trained nurses who are nationals who would care for the population. This is quite serious and needs to be rectified in the near future, taking into consideration that nurses constitute the largest proportion of HRH and deliver the majority of care. Second, the problem of nationalization is relatively more severe in Saudi Arabia and Oman because nationalization among all compared professions falls below the proportion of the country's population of nationals.

The Distribution of Human Resources for Health by Sector

The majority of HRH are employed in the public sector in all GCC states (69 percent on average in the region), except in the United Arab Emirates, where the private sector slightly dominates (making up 55 percent of total HRH counts) (fig. 3.18). Overall, the proportion of HRH in the public sector ranges from a low of 45 percent in the United Arab Emirates to a high of 82 percent in Oman. Having said this, a number of the countries are examining an expanded role for the private sector in delivering and financing healthcare and are exploring viable options for public–private partnerships. Therefore, it is expected that the private sector will be competing more aggressively over HRH in the future, especially if it offers more attractive packages to entice HRH employed in the public sector.

The Distribution of Human Resources for Health by Gender

As seen in figure 3.19, the health workforce in Bahrain, the United Arab Emirates, Oman, and Kuwait is dominated by females—respectively, 77.4 percent, 69.7 percent, 63.8 percent, and 62.0 percent. Only in Saudi Arabia is there a higher proportion of males, with females constituting only 42.1 percent of the health workforce.

However, this figure masks the fact that women still tend to be concentrated in the lower-status health occupations, and to be a minority among more highly trained professions, as seen in the HRH distribution by gender and by professional category in the individual country profiles given above. Particularly, the

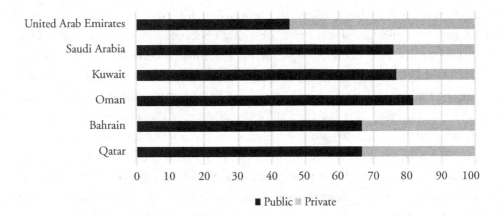

Figure 3.18 **Distribution of Human Resources for Health by Sector in the GCC Countries, 2012**

Sources: Data for Saudi Arabia: Ministry of Health, "Annual Health Statistics Report 2012"; for Oman: Ministry of Health, "Annual Health Report 2012"; for Bahrain: Ministry of Health, Health Information Directorate, "Health Statistics Report 2012"; for United Arab Emirates: "MOH Manpower Statistics 2012"; for Kuwait: "Annual Bulletin of Health Statistics 2012"; for Qatar: "HMC Annual Health Report 2012."

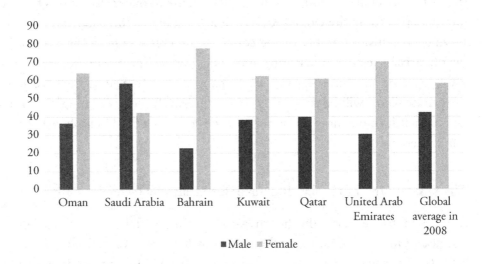

Figure 3.19 **Distribution of Human Resources for Health by Gender in the GCC Countries, 2012**

Sources: Data for Saudi Arabia: Ministry of Health, "Annual Health Statistics Report 2012"; for Oman: Ministry of Health, "Annual Health Report 2012"; for Bahrain: Ministry of Health, Health Information Directorate, "Health Statistics Report 2012"; for United Arab Emirates: "MOH Manpower Statistics 2012"; for Kuwait: "Annual Bulletin of Health Statistics 2012"; for Qatar: "HMC Annual Health Report 2012."

distribution of women by professional category tends to be skewed in favor of nursing and midwifery. Women are, in contrast, poorly represented in other professional categories—such as physicians, dentists, and pharmacists—except in Bahrain, where women dominate all three of these categories.

Beyond the Numbers: The Management of Available Human Resources for Health and Quality Implications

Compensating for HRH shortages to maintain quality of care necessitates optimal use of current resources. However, some GCC states face the issues of segregation of health facilities between citizens and expatriates, restricting certain health facilities to serve nationals only, and thus partially resulting in strenuous workloads for healthcare professionals and exhausting waiting lists for patients.[83] Associated with this concern that further challenges healthcare provision and decision making is the geographical management of HRH, which has prompted officials and residents of certain localities in some GCC states to criticize the allotted HRH and services.[84]

Another, somewhat inevitable, difficulty in providing care results from the expatriate population's many academic backgrounds in HRH and native languages, reaching about 150 languages and dialects in certain countries.[85] Aside from the implications of this diversity for the standard mode of medical practice, proper patient-provider communication is undermined, as is the perceived quality of care by nationals, possibly one factor in the hundreds of millions of dollars being devoted to the treatment of nationals abroad.[86]

Solutions may not always demand the initiation of new strategies. Knowledge sharing provided by a team approach, along with proper monitoring and evaluation by supervisory personnel to ensure that existing strategies and policies are carried out, is an efficient option for improving health outcomes. Implementation and problem solving will require additional training and an increasing focus on quality improvement for all health providers.

LESSONS LEARNED AND RECOMMENDATIONS

The HRH comparison across the GCC states has unearthed a number of common challenges. This section offers key lessons learned, along with associated recommendations.

Opportunity for the Exchange of Expertise and Experiences

At a time when all the GCC states are facing similar challenges, each one of them has had particular successes that can be shared with other countries, along with unsuccessful experiences and initiatives from which other countries may learn. For example, the GCC states can learn from Oman's experience with strategic HRH planning and building educational capacity. The experience of Bahrain, despite its small size, with the nationalization of its workforce is also worth examining. Sharing of experiences allows for cross-fertilization and builds a synergy between system thinkers, planners, and researchers in the various GCC states. In addition to sharing experiences, the sharing of resources may be looked at as well. The unification of efforts and resources entails having certain countries with successful programs fostering and assisting in the implementation of these programs directly in the other GCC states.

Another essential issue is to review the scope of the medical/health educational programs and associated competencies, as well as the practice guidelines, policies, and procedures across the GCC, in order to enhance the options for homogenizing educational programs and the standards of care across the GCC's healthcare systems. This may enhance the region's capacity to share resources as needed, ensure the continuum of patient care across the various countries, and initiate rapid and effective emergency responses during disease outbreaks and spreads, among other positive effects.

The Need to Enhance Human Resources for Health Planning and Forecasting Capacity

There is no doubt that all the GCC states have witnessed exceptionally high growth rates in the number of HRH working in their health sector. Nevertheless, the countries have also realized one of the highest population growth rates reported globally. GCC statistics indicate that, between 2008 and 2011, the populations of Kuwait and Qatar grew by 23 percent and 20 percent, respectively. Such growth is quite challenging to catch up with in terms of the recruitment and distribution of HRH, and the challenge is exacerbated by the strategic vision of enhancing the nationalization of the health workforce.

This challenge means that the GCC states must pool their efforts and consolidate their expertise to devise and test accurate HRH forecasting models that can project HRH needs to guide strategic HRH planning. Such models need to be supported with accurate information, including population growth patterns and demographic transitions, the burden of disease, HRH production capacity, HRH turnover patterns, HRH retirement patterns, and changing consumer/ patient preferences due to increased income.

Furthermore, the GCC states are advised to initiate a policy dialogue to ensure proper alignment between strategic HRH planning and strategic health plans. For example, the emphasis on the importance of primary healthcare to keep the population healthy and delay the onset of disease needs to be supported by an HRH plan that rectifies overspecialization and enhances the proportion of generalists in the HRH workforce. Such actions need to take into consideration profound cultural and societal factors. Before, in the GCC, specializing was seen as professionally unattractive, due to the excessive work hours involved, the patient follow-up needed, and the overall lifestyle associated with a specialty. Now, not going into a specialty is looked on as a sign of incompetence, and it is socially less attractive not to have a specialty or advanced medical degree.

Additionally, each of the GCC states needs to work on analyzing the career trends of HRH, both local and expatriate, to better inform strategic HRH planning and to enhance the recruitment and retention of HRH in local labor markets. Such an analysis should account for all HRH supply channels (graduation from local colleges and universities, enhancing labor market participation, recruiting foreign trained HRH, etc.), as well as the main attrition routes for HRH from the local labor market (turnover, retirement, decreased labor market participation, death, etc.). Analyses should also examine the number and proportion of inactive HRH personnel and the means to draw them back into the labor market.

Insufficient Nationalization of the Workforce

Perhaps the most significant challenge facing the healthcare sector in the GCC states is the nationalization of the workforce. Despite major investments and immense efforts exerted by various countries, the vast majority of the workforce remains nonnational. The issue is exacerbated in the nursing workforce, where three out of six GCC countries (Qatar, the United Arab Emirates, and Kuwait) have severe imbalances, resulting in less than 10 percent of the nursing workforce being local. The issue is also pronounced in the physician workforce, where four of the six GCC states report less than 30 percent of their workforce being local. This is despite the fact that for some countries, the numbers reported are for MOH facilities where the likelihood is high for the employment of nationals. Some might argue that expatriate providers are needed for the high numbers of expatriate populations; but this assumption is erroneous for multiple reasons, the most important of which are

1. The rate of nationalization in some professions falls below the proportion of the country's national population. This is especially true for nurses across the GCC, and could be seen for the other HRH categories in Saudi Arabia and Oman (fig. 3.17).
2. There is a skewed distribution of HRH between the health professions and within the same profession. For instance, the problem of the low proportion of physicians who are nationals out of the total physician workforce in most GCC states is compounded by the overspecialization of physicians who are nationals that does not support staffing needs in primary healthcare centers.
3. The assumption equates between HRH nationals and expatriates in availability, working hours, productivity, and participation in the labor market, which is incorrect in most instances.

The Need to Address Workforce Gender Imbalances

Taking into consideration the GCC region's sociocultural and religious specificity that recommends or mandates that a female be cared for by a practitioner of the same gender, the GCC states need to account in their HRH plans and associated nationalization initiatives for an increase in the proportion of female providers in the healthcare sector. Such initiatives may include facilitating the admission of females into medical studies at the financial, social, and academic levels. Financially, targeted incentives (both monetary and nonmonetary) may be provided to female applicants, especially in professions of great need such as nursing. Socially, media and prominent community figures need to emphasize the importance and contribution of female HRH personnel. And academically, rigorous school curricula are needed to encourage and better equip female and male students alike for an academic track in the health sector. Fostering foreign education opportunities and encouraging volunteer work are other ways to attract females into the HRH professions that may prove to have positive outcomes in the near future.

Furthermore, the instigation of flexible employment modalities can also contribute to enhancing the proportion of female HRH personnel. Indeed, the existing human resource management styles within the examined GCC states are characterized by an evident lack of flexible employment modalities, which may be very much hindering workforce integration as well as reintegration, more so for the female workforce. Modern approaches to effective human resource management have suggested strategies that "nourish retention," and these include but are not limited to offering part-time jobs and job sharing.[87] This is suggested because HRH personnel may prefer to work part time, casually, or for shorter shifts. Moreover, job sharing may give staff members further autonomy in deciding how they will share the position in order to accommodate their lifestyle activities. A study revealed that flexibility in working arrangements is likely to have positive effects on employee health and well-being.[88] Although the casualization of the workforce may increase the number of personnel required to fill each full-time position, this becomes less significant if the total number of staff members retained in the system is increased as a result.

Requiring special attention is the fact that while five of the six GCC states report a female-majority of HRH personnel, this conceals a serious discrepancy in the proportion of female physicians. This proportion remains low, despite the GCC states' efforts to rectify the balance, with the proportion of females in the physician workforce in 2012 subsiding at 28.0 percent, 35.0 percent, and 37.6 percent in Saudi Arabia, Kuwait, and Qatar, respectively. Furthermore, there is a need to identify the HRH professions and specialties where gender sensitivity is critical in order to ensure equitable access to services irrespective of gender. Future plans should, therefore, focus on increasing the proportion of female providers across all specialties, but more specifically within obstetrics and gynecology, family medicine, and pediatrics. Similarly, there is a need to ensure that there are adequate numbers of females among other HRH personnel to properly staff female-only or female sections (a common attribute of healthcare settings in the GCC region) at hospitals and primary healthcare centers.

Future Research Ideas

It is imperative to note that this chapter has focused on analyzing HRH trends within and among the GCC states without scrutinizing the competencies, skills, and expertise of the various types of HRH personnel. Although such an analysis is outside the scope of this chapter, it is essential that it be carried out, not only to assess current and future HRH capacity and shortages but also to decide on in-service training, professional development, and bridging programs that are necessary to equip HRH personnel with the skills needed to serve the needs of the population.

In addition, it would be of great benefit, especially in light of the reported difficulty to recruit experienced HRH personnel, if future examinations could assess the existing recruitment and retention strategies across the GCC states and the means to strengthen them. Furthermore, it is important to assess the practice culture of HRH personnel and whether it adequately supports their well-being, productivity, and retention.

Finally, future studies could examine the HRH configurations that could support healthcare delivery in times of crisis, especially in light of the emerging infectious diseases (Ebola, Corona virus, etc.) and the region's sociopolitical instability.

CONCLUSION

Future HRH plans for the GCC region should build on the efforts reported in recent years, with further investments focused on increasing the ratio of HRH personnel who are nationals, while employing more female providers (especially as physicians). Overall, it is essential for policymakers to take a multisectoral, stakeholder-engaging approach that emphasizes policies relying on accurate statistics and data that are contextualized to the GCC states' sociocultural setting. Furthermore, revisiting certain cultural aspects of the region and properly educating nationals and preparing them with the necessary skills and training are crucial for truly realizing the goals and benefits of nationalization.

NOTES

1. Global Equity Initiative, "Human Resources for Health: Overcoming the Crisis," Harvard University, 2004, www.who.int/hrh/documents/JLi_hrh_report.pdf.

2. S. M. Kabene, C. Orchard, J. Howard, M. Soriano, and R. Leduc, "The Importance of Human Resources Management in Healthcare: A Global Context," *Human Resources for Health* 4, no. 1 (2006): 20; Thomas L. Hall, "Why Plan Human Resources for Health," *Human Resources Development Journal* 2, no. 2 (1998).

3. World Health Organization, "Health Workforce," 2015, www.euro.who.int/en/health-topics/Health-systems/health-workforce/health-workforce.

4. James Campbell, James Buchan, Giorgio Cometto, et al., "Human Resources for Health and Universal Health Coverage: Fostering Equity and Effective Coverage," *Bulletin of the World Health Organization* 91, no. 11 (2013): 853–63; Tomoko Ono, Gaetan Lafortune, and Michael Schoenstein, "Health Workforce Planning in OECD Countries: A Review of 26 Projection Models from 18 Countries," Organization for Economic Cooperation and Development, 2013; Thomas L. Hall, "Why Plan Human Resources for Health," www.who.int/hrh/en/HRDJ_2_2_01.pdf.

5. David E. Guest, Jaap Paauwe, and Patrick Wright, eds., *HRM and Performance Achievements and Challenges* (Chichester, UK: Wiley, 2013); World Health Organization, "Health Workforce."

6. Ibid.

7. Kabene et al., "Importance of Human Resources Management," 20.

8. Lincoln Chen, Timothy Evans, Sudhir Anand, et al., "Human Resources for Health: Overcoming the Crisis," *Lancet* 364, no. 9449 (2004): 1984–90; World Health Organization, "Global Health Observatory: Health Workforce," www.who.int/gho/health_workforce/en/.

9. Ibid.

10. Ibid.

11. Ibid.

12. World Health Organization, "Spotlight on Statistics: A Fact File on Health Workforce Statistics," February 2008, www.who.int/hrh/statistics/spotlight2/en/.

13. Chen et al., "Human Resources."

14. Ibid.

15. World Health Organization, "Working Together for Health: The World Health Report 2006," 2006, www.who.int/whr/2006/whr06_cn.pdf.

16. Najeeb Al-Shorbaji, "E-Health in the Eastern Mediterranean Region: A Decade of Challenges and Achievements," *Eastern Mediterranean Health Journal* 14, special issue (2008): S157–73, http://apps.who.int/iris/bitstream/10665/117599/1/14_s1_s157.pdf.

17. World Health Organization, "Working Together."

18. Fadi El-Jardali, Nuhad Dumit, Diana Jamal, and Gladys Mouro, "Migration of Lebanese Nurses: A Questionnaire Survey and Secondary Data Analysis," *International Journal of Nursing Studies* 45, no. 10 (2008): 1490–1500.

19. Cooperation Council for the Arab States of the Gulf Secretariat General, "The Charter," 2012, www.gccsg.org/eng/indexfe7a.html?action=Sec-Show&TD=1.

20. Information Sector Statistical Department for the GCC Secretariat General, "Gross Domestic Product per Capita," 2012, http://sites.gcc-sg.org/Statistics/.

21. Economist Intelligence Unit, "The GCC in 2020: The Gulf and Its People," 2009, http://graphics.eiu.com/upload/eb/Gulf2020part2.pdf.

22. Information Sector–Statistical Department for the GCC Secretariat General, "Statistical Bulletin," 2012, http://sites.gcc-sg.org/DLibrary/download.php?B=633.

23. Aspen Institute, "Policy Brief for the Global Policy Advisory Council: The Gulf Cooperation Council (GCC) and Health Worker Migration," 2014, www.aspeninstitute.org/sites/default/files/content/images/GCC%20and%20HWM%20Policy%20Brief.pdf; Mona Mourshed, Viktor Hediger, and Toby Lambert, "Gulf Cooperation Council Healthcare: Challenges and Opportunities," World Economic Forum, 2006, www.weforum.org/pdf/Global_Competitiveness_Reports/Reports/chapters/2_1.pdf.

24. Kasim Randeree, "Strategy, Policy, and Practice in the Nationalization of Human Capital: Project Emiratization," *Research and Practice in Human Resource Management* 17, no. 1 (2009): 71.

25. Chen et al., "Human Resources"; Kasim Randeree, "Workforce Nationalization in the Gulf Cooperation Council States," CIRS Occasional Paper 9, Center for International and Regional Studies, Georgetown University School of Foreign Service in Qatar, 2012.

26. Aspen Institute, "Policy Brief for the Global Policy Advisory Council"; Mourshed, Hediger, and Lambert, "Gulf Cooperation Council Healthcare."

27. Aspen Institute, "Policy Brief for the Global Policy Advisory Council."

28. World Health Organization, "Health Workforce," 2014.

29. World Health Organization, "Human Resources Development," 2014.

30. Saudi Arabian Ministry of Health, "Health Statistics Book for the Year 1433," 2013, www.moh.gov.sa/en/Ministry/Statistics/book/Documents/1433.pdf.

31. World Health Organization, *World Health Statistics Report 2013*, 2013, http://apps.who.int/iris/bitstream/10665/82058/1/WHO_HIS_HSI_13.1_eng.pdf?ua=1.

32. Saudi Arabian Ministry of Health, "Health Statistics Book for the Year 1433."

33. Ibid.

34. Saudi Board for Medical Specialization, "Projections of Human Resources for Health in Saudi Arabia," *Almoltaga Alsihi Magazine* 51 (2004): 18.

35. Alpen Capital, "GCC Healthcare Industry," 2014, www.alpencapital.com/downloads/GCC_Healthcare_Sector_22_April_2014_Final.pdf.

36. Oxford Business Group, "Bahrain Continues to See Rapid Growth in the Healthcare Sector," April 15, 2014, www.oxfordbusinessgroup.com/news/bahrain-continues-see-rapid-growth-health-care-sector.

37. Bahrain Ministry of Health, "Health Statistics 2012," 2013, www.moh.gov.bh/PDF/Publications/statistics/HS2012/hs2012_e.htm.

38. Oxford Business Group, "Bahrain Continues to See Rapid Growth."

39. Abdulbari Bener and Ahmed Al Mazroei, "Health Services Management in Qatar," *Croatian Medical Journal* 51, no. 1 (2010): 85–88.

40. Qatar Statistics Authority, "Qatar Social Trends 1998–2010," 2011, www.qsa.gov.qa/eng/publication/pdf-file/Social/Qatar%20Social%20Trends%201998%20-%202010.pdf.

41. Bener and Al Mazroei, "Health Services Management."

42. Qatar Supreme Council of Health, "Qatar Health Report 2012," 2014, www.nhsq.info/app/media/1479.

43. Ibid.

44. Hall, "Why Plan Human Resources for Health."

45. "Officials: Low Salaries, Lack of Training Exacerbate Chronic Shortage of Nurses in Qatar," *Doha News*, October 18, 2012, http://dohanews.co/officials-low-salaries-lack-of-training-exacerbate/.

46. Ibid.

47. Victoria Scott, "Report: Shortage of Qatari Doctors, Nurses to Challenge Health Sector," *Doha News*, January 6, 2014, http://dohanews.co/report-shortage-of-qatari-doctors-nurses-to-challenge-health-sector/.

48. Hamad Medical Corporation, "Annual Report 2013/2014," 2014, www.hmc.org.qa/annualreport2014/pdf/hmc_ar2013_14_en.pdf.

49. Nada Badawi, "Report: Qatar's Healthcare Sector the Fastest Growing in the Region," *Doha News*, April 25, 2014, http://dohanews.co/report-qatars-healthcare-sector-fastest-growing-region/.

50. Supreme Council of Health, "National Health Strategy 2011–2016, Skilled National Workforce," 2014, www.nhsq.info/strategy-goals-and-projects/skilled-national-workforce.

51. Qatar Statistical Authority, "Annual Abstract 2012: Health Services Chapter," 2014, www.qsa.gov.qa/eng/GeneralStatistics.htm#Annual_Abstract_2014.

52. Supreme Council of Health, "Qatar Health Report 2012."

53. Ibid.

54. Kuwait Ministry of Health, "Kuwait Health Indicators: Monitoring Health Situation, Trends and Health System Performance, 2012–2013," 2014.

55. Kuwait Central Statistical Bureau, "Annual Bulletin of the Health Statistics 2012," 2013, www.csb.gov.kw/Socan_Statistic_EN.aspx?ID=59.

56. Ben Garcia, "Few Arabs Take Up Nursing as a Career," *Kuwait Times*, March 22, 2014.

57. Ibid.

58. Kuwait Ministry of Health, "Kuwait Health Indicators."

59. Khaled F. Al-Jarallah, Mohamed A. Moussa, and Khadija Figen Al-Khanfar, "The Physician Workforce in Kuwait to the Year 2020," *International Journal of Health Planning and Management* 25, no. 1 (2010): 49–62; Kuwait Ministry of Health, "Health, Kuwait XLIX," no. 49 (2010).

60. Peter Brooks, Helen M. Lapsley, and David Butt, "Medical Workforce Issues in Australia: 'Tomorrow's Doctors-Too Few, Too Far,'" *Medical Journal of Australia* 179, no. 4 (2003): 206; US Department of Health and Human Services, "Physician Supply and Demand: Projections to 2020," 2006, http://bhpr.hrsa.gov/healthworkforce/supplydemand/medicine/physician2020 projections.pdf.

61. Khaled F. Al-Jarallah and Mohamed A. Moussa, "Specialty Choices of Kuwaiti Medical Graduates during the Last Three Decades," *Journal of Continuing Education in the Health Professions* 23, no. 2 (2003): 94–100.

62. K. Al-Jarallah, M. Moussa, and K. F. Al-Khanfar, "The Physician Workforce in Kuwait to the Year 2020," www.ncbi.nlm.nih.gov/pubmed/19784937.

63. Alpen Capital, "GCC Healthcare Industry," 2014, www.alpencapital.com/industry-reports.html.

64. Neil Churchill, "UAE Needs 13,000 Doctors by 2014," *Gulf Business*, 2012, http://gulfbusiness.com/2012/06/uae-needs-13000-doctors-by-2014/#.VUoHZpSUfiQ.

65. Ibid.

66. Manal Ismail, "Abu Dhabi to Increase Doctor Numbers by 40%," *The National*, 2012; Sananda Sahoo, "Shortage of Healthcare Workers in the UAE Fuels Poaching and Cost Increases," *The National*, 2013, www.thenational.ae/uae/hospitals/shortage-of-healthcare-workers-in-the-uae-fuels-poaching-and-cost-increases.

67. Ismail, "Abu Dhabi to Increase Doctor Numbers."

68. Colliers International, "United Arab Emirates: Healthcare Overview, Q4 2013," 2013, www.colliers.com/-/media/CF692F58BA4D44A08D55FE7F1E54E584.ashx?la=en-GB; Sahoo, "Shortage of Healthcare Workers."

69. Colliers International, "United Arab Emirates."

70. Ismail, "Abu Dhabi to Increase Doctor Numbers."

71. Colliers International, "United Arab Emirates."

72. Jennifer Bell, "Lack of Emirati Doctors Is 'Worrying Problem,' Middle East Health Leaders Told," *The National*, January 28, 2014.

73. Moeness Alshishtawy, "Medical Specialties in Oman: Scaling Up through National Action," *Oman Medical Journal* 24, no. 4 (2009): 279–87.

74. Ibid.

75. Alpen Capital, "GCC Healthcare Industry," 2014, www.alpencapital.com/downloads/GCC_Healthcare_Sector_22_April_2014_Final.pdf.

76. Cleofe Maceda, "Healthcare Sector in GCC Faces Talent Shortage," *Gulf News*, January 10, 2014, http://gulfnews.com/business/sectors/careers/health-care-sector-in-gcc-faces-talent-shortage-1.1275896; Scott, "Report."

77. MEED, "Healthcare Strategies in the Gulf 2014," April 23, 2014, www.meed.com/research/healthcare-strategies-in-the-gulf-2014/3191410.article.

78. Kate Emery, "Healthcare in the Middle East," Care Visions International Recruitment, March 19, 2012.

79. Maceda, "Healthcare Sector in GCC Faces Talent Shortage."

80. Ibid.; Vesela Todorova, "Shortage of Healthcare Professionals in GCC as Demand Set

to Soar 240% in 20 Years," *The National*, January 5, 2014, www.thenational.ae/uae/health /shortage-of-healthcare-professionals-in-gcc-as-demand-set-to-soar-240-in-20-years.

81. MEED, "Healthcare Strategies."

82. Statistical Department for the GCC Secretariat General, "Statistical Bulletin 2013," 2013; D. Al-Buainain, S. Al-Muraikhi, S. Al-Humoud, and H. Al-Malki, "Women and Men in the State of Qatar: A Statistical Profile 2012," No. 99921-35-75, 2013, Supreme Council of Family Affairs and Qatar Statistics Authority; J. Snoj, "Population of Qatar by Nationality," *Bq Magazine*, 2013, www.bqdoha.com/2013/12/population-qatar; World Bank, "Qatar World Development Indicators," 2014.

83. Azmat Haroon, "Health Center Move Irks Many Families," *The Peninsula*, May 18, 2012, http://thepeninsulaqatar.com/news/qatar/194776/health-centre-move-irks-many -families.

84. "Councilors Lament Shortage of Medical Services in Their Areas," *The Peninsula*, September 3, 2014, http://thepeninsulaqatar.com/news/qatar/298584/councillors-lament -shortage-of-medical-services-in-their-areas.

85. Qatar Supreme Council of Health, "Caring for the Community: Qatar's Leading Role in Combatting a Global Epidemic," *Qatar Health: Magazine of the Supreme Council of Health* 5 (2014): 34, www.nhsq.info/app/media/1393.

86. Supreme Council of Health, Hamad Medical Corporation, and Primary Healthcare Corporation, "National Health Strategy 2011–2016," 2011, www.cf.am/files/news/167/b32e2 ddf31eaf7a.pdf; Supreme Council of Health, "Qatar National Health Accounts Report, 2012," www.sch.gov.qa/home-en.

87. Betty R. Kupperschmidt, "Multi-Generation Employees: Strategies for Effective Management," *Healthcare Manager* 19, no. 1 (2000): 65–76.

88. K. Joyce, R. Pabayo, J. A. Critchley, and C. Bambra, "Flexible Working Conditions and Their Effects on Employee Health and Wellbeing," February 17, 2010, www.cochrane.org/CD 008009/PUBHLTH_flexible-working-conditions-and-their-effects-on-employee-health-and -wellbeing.

4

MENTAL HEALTH IN THE GULF COOPERATION COUNCIL STATES

Suhaila Ghuloum and Hassen Al-Amin

The indigenous populations of the countries overlooking the Gulf share a common language, religion, historical background, culture, and, to a large extent, a similar economic profile. These commonalities culminated in the 1981 formation of the Gulf Cooperation Council (GCC), which consists of Qatar, Kuwait, Bahrain, Saudi Arabia, Oman, and the United Arab Emirates.

Across the GCC, economic booms—starting with the discovery of oil, and, more lately, of natural gas in Qatar—have resulted in vast and rapid developmental plans and changes to the infrastructure in these countries. Qatar, the United Arab Emirates, and the GCC's other members are now hosting international sports, politics, and other cultural events. All these plans require manpower and expertise that are either insufficient locally or not available at all. Subsequently, there has been a rise in the population of the GCC's member states and a change in its ethnic composition. In 2013 the GCC's total population was nearly 50 million. Since 2007 its compound annual growth rate has been 4 percent, among the highest in the world.[1] This is largely attributed to the influx of expatriate workers and the region's high birthrate. Particularly notable among the various ambitious endeavors in these countries are their considerable plans for healthcare advancement. The healthcare needs of this population have exceeded the current service capacity, resulting in regional plans to build more hospitals. Saudi Arabia, Qatar, and the United Arab Emirates are in the middle of a hospital construction boom. The healthcare sector in the GCC will rise to $56 billion by 2020.[2] Healthcare in the GCC is largely government subsidized, and the private insurance sector has been introduced only recently in some of the member states. However, for the citizens of these countries, healthcare is provided free of charge.

The Health Ministers Council of the Arab Countries in the Gulf was established in 1976. In 1991 it was renamed the Executive Board of the Health Ministers for the Arab Gulf Cooperation Countries. This Executive Board includes Qatar, Kuwait, Saudi Arabia, Bahrain, the United Arab Emirates, and Oman. Yemen joined in 2003. The board's main goal is to achieve cooperation and integration in health services between the GCC states. Its mission includes promoting coordination between member states in preventive, treatment, and rehabilitation efforts; the dissemination of knowledge; and setting unified priorities for healthcare while sharing experiences through regular meetings and training opportunities.

The Executive Board supervises the work of several committees that cover a number of healthcare priorities and aim to unify standards of care as well as purchasing practices. For instance, the Gulf executive plan for improving mental health is a five-year plan formed by the Gulf Mental Health Committee for the period 2011–16.[3] The plan describes ten strategies, with time frames and indicators for implementation. The following is a summary of these strategies:

- Organizing services in mental healthcare where the emphasis is on the need for mental health representation in the organizational structure of the ministries of health (MOHs), including an assigned budget, job descriptions for employees in mental health, and community mental health services. It also highlights the importance of a national committee for mental health.
- Strengthening mental health delivery in primary care, with training opportunities and management guidelines for primary care physicians on mental health issues.
- Recognizing vulnerable groups and prioritizing services that target them. These include mothers, children, and adolescents; substance misuse; and the existence of a mental health disaster-management protocol and plan.
- Improving information technology and facilitating the exchange of information between GCC members.
- Improving legislation and policies. The aim is for each member state to have a mental health law that also addresses the rights of people with a mental illness.
- Human resource development, where the focus is on continuous professional development and training opportunities for all disciplines.
- Improving budget and funding programs. The plan specifies a mental

health budget, to be set at a minimum of 5 percent of the total health budget allocation.

- Quality improvement projects. This initiative encourages all mental health facilities in the GCC to receive a recognized accreditation, have a sentinel event annual report, and have at least one major quality improvement project per year.
- Mental health promotion and education that emphasize the need for an assigned entity responsible for mental health promotion and awareness; and the presence of awareness activities or campaigns.

The plan outlines broad principles, but the details of implementation are left to each member state to decide according to its individual needs and system preferences.

THE PREVALENCE OF MENTAL ILLNESS

The prevalence of mental illness has been reported only for some countries in the GCC, primarily the United Arab Emirates and more recently Qatar. Data on its prevalence among the elderly and youth are almost nonexistent.

In a prevalence survey in Qatar using the Composite International Diagnostic Interview, which uses ICD-10 and DSM-IV diagnostic criteria, the most common disorder among the Qatari population was generalized anxiety disorder (20.4 percent), followed by major depression (19.1 percent) and social phobia (17.03 percent). The majority was in the mild to moderate degree of symptom severity. Prevalence was higher in women for generalized anxiety disorder, depression, social phobias, and specific phobias. The thirty-day functioning measure was worse in women as compared with men, reflecting a higher impact of disease on women.[4]

The results indicate that one in five of the population will develop a form of mental illness at any one time. Three of the top five causes of disability and three of the six highest disease burdens in Qatar are related to mental health. Furthermore, psychiatric disorders account for more than 25 percent of the disease burden in Qatar, accounting for 79,890 total disability-adjusted life years.[5]

Interestingly, during the screening process, questions related to suicidal ideation or attempts and substance misuse were unanimously denied; the total score on these questions was zero. This reflects the higher stigma associated with self-harm and drug misuse, partly because of the religious implications of both.

Drug intake and attempts to end life are considered *haram* (against Islamic principles) and are attached to strong social taboos. However, substance misuse is one of the top causes of disability and burdens of disease in Qatar. Suicide in this region is underreported, and often is not documented as the cause of death on death certificates. The true prevalence is still expected to be quite low because of religious and social factors. Furthermore, self-harm attempts have legal implications and are thus also underreported or denied. By legislation, cases of self-harm attempts must be reported to the police. In Qatar this is done through the Emergency Department as the point of first presentation. Although criminal charges are never pressed for self-harming, an investigation is often conducted, primarily to exclude homicidal possibility. The ordeal and fear of consequences of police involvement mean that the majority of cases deny suicidal intention and claim an accidental overdose. Those who are aware of the system avoid it by going to private hospitals, where reporting does not occur, or opt not to present for medical care. The underreported prevalence of self-harm has negative influences on service planning, prioritizing, and preventive efforts. Preliminary data gathered by the authors for Qatar, not yet published, report 48 cases of suicide in one year for a population of almost 1.5 million; these cases mostly occurred among the South Asian residents of the country, hanging being the most common method by far.[6] This is comparable to the prevalence in their relevant country of origin. Among those presenting with attempted suicide, a drug overdose was the most common method, primarily with East Asian Muslims of unskilled occupations.

MENTAL HEALTH SERVICES

Mental health services in the GCC remain largely hospital-based, with negligible community-based facilities and outreach or rehabilitation programs (table 4.1). These statistics vary widely, perhaps related to the validity of the underlying data or to differences in defining particular health facilities or clinics in each of the countries. The emphasis until recently was on building large institutions away from the general hospital facilities, with scarce residential or medium- to long-term rehabilitation or vocational settings. Mental health was not seen as a priority area in the health strategies of any of the GCC states, and consequently funding was minimal. These services primarily target an adult population, with fewer resources for youth and the elderly. There is a lack of specialized in-patient facilities for adolescents or specialized mother and baby units. Subspecialty services for adults have yet to be developed. The population in the GCC is gener-

Table 4.1   **Summary of Mental Health Services per 100,000 Population in the GCC States**

Variable	Qatar	Kuwait	Bahrain	Saudi Arabia	Oman	United Arab Emirates
Beds in mental hospitals	3.98	32.78	28.0	11.43	2.20	1.7
Beds in general hospitals	0.00	0.00	0.00	0.38	0.41	0.53
Day treatment facilities	0.13	0.03	0.25	0.01	0.00	0.00
Beds in community residential facilities	0.99	Unknown	—	0.91	0.00	0.00
Admissions to mental hospitals	3.98	85.23	129.22	76.53	27.16	7.01
Treatment in psychiatry outpatient facilities	990	Unknown	Unknown	Unknown	360.26	220.1

Source: Data from World Health Organization, Atlas of Global Health for 2011.

ally considered "young." In Oman the mean age of the population is 18.8 years.[7] In Qatar the proportion of people above the age of sixty-five years is less than 1 percent. This is explained by the high influx of foreign workforce members required to achieve the infrastructure needed for the Qatar National Vision 2030. Single male laborers represent the vast majority of this foreign workforce. In addition, the particular needs of this population have yet to be addressed. The effects of immigration, living conditions, and financial and social stressors should also be taken into consideration when planning the mental health services in each of the GCC states.

The GCC states' clinical care most commonly follows the guidelines established in the United Kingdom, the United States, and Canada. There is a gap in the availability of culture-specific assessment scales and culturally based treatment guidelines. The available screening or measurement tools (e.g., psychometric testing) are mainly translated tools that have not necessarily been validated for the specific treated population. We are actively working now to validate and culturally adapt the most commonly used assessment tools using rigorous scientific research methods.

International best practice suggests that most people with mental illness can be treated in the community. In the GCC primary care plays a minor role in the care of patients with mental illness, and the system relies heavily on psychiatric hospital outpatient clinics to provide the care needed by all patients, including those with a high prevalence of disorders such as depression and anxiety.

Mental health clinics are established in some primary healthcare centers in Saudi Arabia. There are only a few community-based psychiatric in-patient facilities that provide residential care and where supervision is essentially provided by nurses and support staff. Primary healthcare center clinicians have little training in mental health and have restricted prescribing privileges for psychotropic medications.[8] The same applies to most of the GCC, where the majority of physicians in primary care are general practitioners and where a smaller number of family physicians receive some training in psychiatry as part of their training program. Bahrain and Oman have better services at the primary care level, with a pathway for referring patients to and from the psychiatry hospital and with treatment guidelines available at primary care centers.

The primary care system in Qatar is evolving with regard to mental healthcare. Identified physicians are currently receiving training in the management of mental illness, with a focus on depression and anxiety disorders, given that they are the most prevalent ones. The mental health plan stipulates establishing a number of community-based mental health facilities adjacent to primary care centers. This ensures more accessible and acceptable facilities for the population, and allows for better communication with the adjacent primary care centers for the benefit of referred patients. The anticipated role for primary care centers includes screening and thus early identification of people with mental health issues. It is well established that early recognition and intervention result in better outcomes and enhance recovery.

The mental health services in Qatar, Kuwait, Bahrain, and Oman are centralized, with one governmental hospital providing the service for the whole population with minimal coverage from the private sector. The United Arab Emirates and Saudi Arabia have a number of regional hospitals, and the private sector is slightly larger in scale compared with the other GCC states. In Qatar there are only four private psychiatrists, two of which are within a private general hospital. All are based in Doha, with no private in-patient facility. Current service utilization in Qatar is estimated at 25 percent of the need for Qataris, and only 5 percent of the need for non-Qataris. Although data are not readily available, these figures were based on the prevalence data and the number of patients attending the psychiatry department.

For mental health, the projected increase in the demand for services is estimated at 240 percent by 2025. The projected growth in demand for hospital beds across the GCC by 2025 averages 140 percent, with the highest growth affecting the United Arab Emirates, followed by Saudi Arabia, and the least in Bahrain. Qatar will a see 100 percent increase in demand.[9] It is doubtful whether the current reliance on the public sector in the GCC can be sustained to provide services, given this sharp increase in demand. There is a need to shift the focus of care from the government to the private sector.

POLICIES AND LEGISLATION

Table 4.2 summarizes the status of policies and services in mental health for the GCC. In the past few years, all member states, apart from the United Arab Emirates, have developed mental health plans, which are at varying stages of implementation. Statistics on the percentage of gross domestic product spent on health are available for Qatar, Bahrain, and Saudi Arabia; all are less than 4 percent, in contrast to the global figure of 6 percent. Under the direction of the Gulf executive plan for improving mental health, a mental health law was drafted in each member state, sharing the same broad principles of care and highlighting the rights of patients with mental illness. The law also mandates a supervisory authority to oversee the implementation of the law and addresses any breaches of patients' rights, according to the system in each GCC country. In Saudi Arabia a human rights committee is responsible for overseeing inspections of mental health facilities to ensure that patients' rights are respected and preserved. However, this is an ad hoc committee formulated in response to complaints rather than a standing committee. No similar system exists in the rest of the GCC. The laws remain drafts, awaiting approval. However, in Qatar the law has been revised and approved by the cabinet, and will shortly be recognized officially.

Consumer associations are present in some countries, mainly Saudi Arabia, Kuwait, and Bahrain, and very recently in Qatar. Although they are active in efforts to raise awareness, these associations are not involved in service planning or development, with the exception of Bahrain. In fact, most of these associations are advocacy groups not composed of service users.

Qatar's national mental health strategy, Changing Minds, Changing Lives, was launched in 2013. The five-year strategy was endorsed by Her Highness Sheikha Moza bint Nasser "to deliver the best possible care for those affected by mental illness, care that is high quality, culturally appropriate, and accessible." The vision is to provide "good mental health and well-being for the people of Qatar, supported by integrated mental health services with access to the right care, at the right time, in the right place."[10]

Table 4.2   **Summary of Mental Health Policy and Legislation in the GCC States**

Variable	Qatar	Kuwait	Bahrain	Saudi Arabia	Oman	UAE
Total health expenditures as % of GDP	2.46	3.31	4.54	4.97	3.02	2.81
Mental health policy	Yes	Yes	Yes	Yes	Yes	No
Mental health plan	Yes	Yes	Yes	Yes	Yes	Yes
Mental health law	In process	No	In process	Yes	In process	Yes
Mental health expenditures as % of total health budget	1.95	—	3.96	3.89	—	—
Primary care mental health services	In process	Yes	Yes	Partial	Yes	In process

Source: Data from World Health Organization, *Atlas of Global Health for 2011.*

The strategy is reflected in a mental health plan that highlights four objectives: mental health promotion and prevention, integrated and comprehensive mental health services, strengthening leadership and governance, and promoting research that translates into evidence-based practice. These objectives are aligned with the World Health Organization's Global Action Plan initiative, and with the GCC's mental health strategic plan.

AWARENESS AND PROMOTION

Mental health literacy in the GCC region is a challenge. The lack of awareness about mental illness and the high stigma associated with it, with very common misconceptions, result in delayed help-seeking behavior. Patients often seek help late in the course of illness, after they have exhausted the traditional healing methods available both locally and regionally. And patients often resort to psychiatric help when their condition deteriorates and affects functioning, or when the patient presents a danger to self or others, thus necessitating admission. Often, families encourage patients to discontinue their treatment once the acuity has subsided, ultimately resulting in further relapses and complicating the management. Like all diseases, mental illness carries a better prognosis with early intervention and treatment.

A cross-sectional review of the prevalence of mental illness among visitors to faith healers in Riyadh, using the Mini International Neuropsychiatric Interview (MINI 6.0), showed that 34.9 percent of subjects had depressive disorder, 18.7

percent had anxiety disorders, and 6.9 percent had psychotic disorder. The practices used by the faith healers in providing treatment included reading verses from the Holy Quran, or using water and olive oil blessed by reciting the Holy Quran over them. Some patients (4.4 percent) also reported the use of beating, choking, or electrical shocks as methods of intervention.[11]

In Qatar a cross-sectional survey of the knowledge, attitudes, and perceptions of Arab residents regarding mental illness showed that 48.3 percent believe mental illness is a punishment from God, 38.7 percent interpret it as possession by evil spirits, and 39.2 percent believe it is treatable with traditional healers. Still, 53.5 percent thought patients with mental illness are dangerous, and 40.6 percent confused mental illness with mental retardation. In the same survey, 28.6 percent described feelings of shame to have a family member with mental illness. For the majority (64.2 percent), the media were the source of information. On a positive note, 83.7 percent reported that patients could be treated with psychotherapy; this might have significant implications, especially now that care in the region is largely psychopharmacological.[12]

RESEARCH, TRAINING, AND EDUCATION

Overall health research in the GCC has increased during the past decade, with more funding resources becoming available. The creation of the Qatar Foundation for Education, Science, and Community Development provides a considerable source of funding to facilitate health research in Qatar and the region, in collaboration with researchers from Qatar. However, mental health research remains inadequate and insufficient. In a PubMed review of mental health research publications from the GCC, a total of 192 publications were found over a twenty-year period from 1989 to 2008. This represents less than 1 percent of the GCC's biomedical research. The majority was epidemiological in nature.[13] Afifi conducted a Medline review of mental health publications in the Arab world and found that 37 percent were from Kuwait and Saudi Arabia, largely focusing on substance misuse and depressive disorders.[14]

Although residency training programs have been established for physicians specializing in mental health, those seeking to train other clinical staff working in mental health facilities face many challenges. This workforce is composed largely of expatriates with varying educational and language backgrounds, and the majority are not trained primarily in mental health. The presence of medical and nursing colleges allows for enhanced teaching opportunities for these specialties. The presence of international schools—such as Weill Cornell

Medicine–Qatar, the University of Calgary's Nursing School and the College of the North Atlantic in Qatar, and the Royal College of Surgeons in Bahrain, as well as international healthcare providers (e.g., Johns Hopkins in the United Arab Emirates)—will help to improve the educational experience and build the region's research potential. The opening of Weill Cornell Medicine–Qatar and the inception of student clerkships in the psychiatry department have been reflected in the training standards of the residents involved in their supervision and education.

The drive to acquire international accreditation for hospitals has also contributed to the enhancement of the care provided. Examples include the Joint Commission International for international facilities including hospitals, and the Accreditation Council for Graduate Medical Education International (ACGME-I) for international physician residency training programs—created by the United States–based Accreditation Council for Graduate Medical Education, which accredits residency programs in the United States. These accreditations, though initially faced with resistance and opposition from clinicians accustomed to certain methods of practice, have in fact encouraged the revision of the practice policies and procedures. Such revisions would ultimately facilitate the achievement of the highest standards of patient safety and improve the training standards of clinicians. The ACGME-I's accreditation meant an overhaul of the training programs, with a focus on junior doctors acquiring competencies in clinical practice with graded levels of supervision that would prepare them for independent safe practice. Within the GCC states, the United Arab Emirates, Qatar, and Oman have received ACGME-I accreditation for their training programs.[15]

SHARED CHALLENGES

The biggest challenge facing implementation of the GCC's mental health plan is the stigma to which mental illness is subjected. Although this stigma is a worldwide issue, it is notably higher in this part of the world, and often presents a major obstacle to help-seeking behaviors. Access to care is more likely to be delayed until there are acute presentations, and noncompliance with the management plan hinders recovery. Stigma is found not only among the general public; policymakers and decision makers are equally affected, and more efforts are needed to improve awareness at every level and thus to ensure that mental health gets the attention it deserves. The lack of data makes this task even harder. We need to reflect through data the impact of mental illness on society, the burden of illness in this region, and the impaired quality of life resulting from the existing shortage of rehabilitation- and recovery-based programs. Among clinicians, we need to reflect, through research evidence, the prevalence of mental illness in the context of other conditions—for example, cardiovascular disease, diabetes, and cancer—and the detrimental effects of untreated depression on the management and outcome of these physical illnesses.

Although Qatar is fortunate to have funding resources for research through the Qatar Foundation's National Priorities Research Program and the Hamad Medical Corporation's research budget, this is not true for its GCC neighbors. Attempts to collaborate on research are faced with significant bureaucratic obstacles. A clear research strategy that highlights the key priority areas for each country will ensure that the needs are being addressed with the proper research methods.

The lack of undergraduate educational programs in specialties related to mental health—such as occupational therapy, clinical psychology, nursing, and mental health social work—increases reliance on the foreign workforce, which is not always culturally competent, and thus jeopardizes the therapeutic alliance and treatment outcomes. There is a need for a workforce development strategy that addresses the local workforce's current challenges and includes training initiatives. Although there are clear plans in the region to develop subspecialties in mental health service provision, the care of adults with learning disabilities remains overlooked, and more resources should be available for them.

A broader challenge shared by the GCC states is the impact of their rapidly transitioning societies on the mental health of their youth populations. Although society at large remains attached to its traditional values, young people are more exposed to social media and other means of access to ideologies that are very different from their society's norms. The generation gap between parents and their children is very wide, and we are beginning to see youth with social and religious conflicts that affect their sense of belonging to society, their communication with their family members of an older generation, and their own mental health. As women are becoming more aware of their rights, their role in society is changing, as are their expectations of their roles within family. Muslim men are allowed more than one wife, which is a practice quite common in this region and one that was previously considered "acceptable" by many women. However, colloquial reports suggest that women are now less likely to accept polygamy, though they may still opt to continue in such a married status for social reasons. The mental health consequences of these changes have not been studied.

As the region develops, and society's composition changes, the health demands of this rapidly increasing population need to be met. For mental health services, the demand exceeds the service availability. The highest population increase has been in single male laborers. Many of these workers have left their country for the first time, are not familiar with the language or culture of this region, and may not be familiar with the type of work offered to them. Their living conditions may be suboptimal and may not provide privacy. All these factors result in many workers showing symptoms of adjustment- and stress-related disorders or acute psychotic presentations. In Qatar these cases are responsible for almost 30 percent of the psychiatry bed occupancy. Although this is a shared challenge among the GCC states, there is a scarcity of research to further evaluate the situation. The available literature mainly consists of theoretical presentations and clinical reports.[16] Many workers deny a past psychiatric history for fear of losing their jobs. Efforts need to be made to ensure that mental health support and counseling are provided to them early on, at accessible locations, to prevent the development of mental illness.

The ministers of health of all its member states endorsed the GCC's mental health plan, with a commitment to its implementation. Rapid developments are occurring in each of these countries in clinical, educational, and research areas. The region is investing in its local population to receive high-quality undergraduate or postgraduate training, both locally and internationally. We will see a mental healthcare workforce accustomed to evidence-based practice, conducting research to provide better data and culture-specific clinical care, and committed to educating junior clinicians. The clinical care is shifting away from the paternalistic model to one that engages patients and their families or caregivers in the treatment plan. Efforts to raise public awareness are being made, to varying degrees.

Primary care will adopt the role of screening for mental illness, managing the high prevalence of disorders and the stable patients with chronic mental illness in close collaboration with the psychiatrists at the tertiary facilities. Patients' rights will be preserved and regulated through legislation, while the care of patients will be personalized and evidence based. Mental health services will be integrated with the other medical and social services, with a focus on recovery and reintegration into the community. The latter would also require a commitment to implement preventive methods, early recognition, proper interventions, and accessible services.

NOTES

1. FALAK Consulting, "GCC Health Care—A Diagnosis: Expanding Horizons for a Healthy Future," Industry Research, 2014.

2. Ibid.

3. Gulf Mental Health Committee, "Gulf Executive Plan for Improving Mental Health," Riyadh, 2011.

4. Suhaila Ghuloum, Abdulbari Bener, Elnour E. Dafeeah, Tariq Al-Yazidi, Ahmed ElAmin Mustapha, and Ahmed E. Zakareia. "Lifetime Prevalence of Common Mental Disorders in Qatar: Using WHO Composite International Diagnostic Interview (WHO-CIDI)," *International Journal of Clinical Psychiatry and Mental Health* 2 (2014): 38–46.

5. Institute for Health Metrics and Evaluation, *Global Burden of Disease: Generating Evidence, Guiding Policy* (Seattle: University of Washington, 2010).

6. S. Ghuloum and Hassen Alamin, "Prevalence of Suicide and Suicidal Behavior in Qatar," unpublished research data.

7. Sanjay Jaju, Samir Al-Adawi, and Asya Al-Riyami, "Prevalence and Age-of-Onset Distributions of DSM IV Mental Disorders and Their Severity among Schoolgoing Omani Adolescents and Youths: WMH-CIDI Findings," *Child and Adolescent Psychiatry and Mental Health* 3 (2009): 29.

8. Naseem Akhtar Qureshi, Abdulhameed Abdullah Al-Habeeb, and Harold G. Koenig, "Mental Health System in Saudi Arabia: An Overview," *Neuropsychiatric Disease and Treatment* 9 (2013): 1121–35.

9. Mona Mourshed, Victor Hediger, and Toby Lambert, "Gulf Cooperation Council Health Care: Challenges and Opportunities," in *Global Competitiveness Report*, ed. World Economic Forum (Geneva: World Economic Forum, 2007).

10. General Secretariat, Supreme Council of Health, State of Qatar, "Qatar Mental Health Strategy: Changing Minds, Changing Lives, 2013–2018."

11. Fahad D. Alosaimi, Youssef Alshehri, Ibrahim Alfraih, Ayedh Alghamdi, Saleh Aldahash, Haifa Alkhuzayem, and Haneen Albeeeshi, "The Prevalence of Psychiatric Disorders among Visitors to Faith Healers in Saudi Arabia," *Pakistan Journal of Medical Science* 30, no. 5 (2014): 1077–82.

12. A. Bener and S. Ghuloum, "Gender Differences in Knowledge, Attitude, and Practice towards Mental Illness in a Rapidly Developing Arab Society," *International Journal of Social Psychiatry*, June 30, 2010.

13. O. T. Osman and M. Afifi, "Troubled Minds in the Gulf: Mental Health Research in the United Arab Emirates (1989-2008),"*Asia Pacific Journal of Public Health* 22, no. 3 (suppl. 2010): 48S–53S.

14. M. M. Afifi, "Analysis of Mental Health Publications from Arab Countries in PubMed, 1987–2002," *Neurosciences (Riyadh)* 9, no. 2 (2004): 113–18.

15. See www.acgme-i.org/News-and-Announcements/ACGME-I-Data-Book/ArticleID /185/2015-2016-ACGME-I-Data-Resource-Book.

16. Maha Al-Ghafry, Marwa Saleh, and Ziad Kronfol, "Mental Health Issues among Migrant Workers in the Gulf Cooperation Council Countries: Literature Review and Case Illustrations," *Qatar Foundation Annual Research Forum Proceedings*, 2012.

SUBSTANCE ABUSE IN THE GULF COOPERATION COUNCIL STATES

Samir Al-Adawi

The unique geographical location, economic profile, and demography of the Gulf region provide an interesting background for examining whether the global challenge of abuse of mind-altering substances has encroached on this region. In terms of its geography, it is located close to what is termed the Golden Crescent or Drug Belt—countries in Southeast Asia that are notorious for their regular bumper crop production and use of drugs. Furthermore, being a hub for international trade and transshipment, and with its large influx of contract workers from different parts of the world, the countries that constitute the Gulf Cooperation Council (GCC) could be an amalgamation of cultures, trades, and individuals that could act as a background for the proliferation of drug trafficking and its consumptions.[1] Economically, the GCC has been acclaimed as the fastest-growing economy, stemming from its revenue from the exploration of oil and natural gas coupled with booming real estate and international trade sectors. With a large bulk of the world's oil reserves located in the GCC, the oil boom resulted in a rapidly growing economy and in an amassing of wealth in the region.

The GCC has been applauded with a qualitative leap in its quality of life. It has been credited as having "very high" (Qatar, Saudi Arabia, the United Arab Emirates, Bahrain, and Kuwait) and "high" (Oman) human development, according to the United Nations Development Program.[2] The GCC thrived, and thus achieved most of the eight Millennium Development Goals—international development goals for 2015 that were set in 2010 by the United Nations, which all its member states were committed to reach.[3] On the educational front, the GCC has instituted an educational program that has eradicated illiteracy;

however, there is concern regarding this educational approach and performance.[4] Most of the GCC spends a significant share of its gross national product to furnish universal education for its citizens. Illiteracy is on the wane, as educational institutions have spread to all corners of the region, and concerted efforts are under way to improve the existing gender gap,[5] as women are "showing tenacity in making efforts to surmount the barriers" of the gap.[6]

The region's improved standard of living in recent decades has coincided with the baby boom[7] and presented some challenges in safeguarding the welfare of a rapidly acculturating population.[8] The spread of education may have sparked an urban drift, whereby youth may find little sense of belonging in their society.[9] According to Al-Barwani and Albeelyb,[10] there is a public concern for weakening of family ties in the region as children are left on their own due to increased activity of women outside the house and thereby setting the background for "proximal abandonment," as reported in the psychological literature.[11] The empowerment of women has improved in some of the GCC states; Oman, for example, has opened the door for Omani women to join the workforce.[12] The GCC is characterized by a youth bulge, given that the bulk of its population is under the age of thirty years.[13] The increase in population means that the number of people afflicted with maladjustments is likely to increase. There are indications elsewhere that some vulnerable youth may be led to self-medication with detrimental substances, or be involved in risky behavior that may have an adverse long-term effect on themselves and society.[14] Therefore, concerted efforts are needed to examine the prevailing trend in the use of mind-altering substances in the GCC, and therefore enlightened views toward harm reduction could be contemplated as well as allocating resources for evidence-based interventions as a means of reducing the burden of mind-altering substances.

Mind-altering substances and their aftermath—addiction—have been variously perceived as the "scourge" of humankind since time immemorial, though some societies appeared to condone it, whereas others upheld puritanical attitudes toward such addiction.[15] The terms "substance abuse" and "drug abuse" have been recently replaced by the term "substance use disorder," which refers to the use of one or more substances leading to a clinically significant impairment or distress.[16] The *Diagnostic and Statistical Manual of Mental Disorders IV (DSM-IV)* provided separate categories for substance abuse and substance dependence. However, the new version of diagnosis nomenclature, *DSM-V*, has clustered demarcation between "substance abuse" and "substance dependence." The new category is titled "substance use disorders."[17] In this chapter, these terms are used interchangeably. Various compounds have been linked to trigger substance use disorder, including alcohol, tobacco, caffeine and methylxanthines, cannabis, hallucinogens, inhalants, opioids, sedatives, hypnotics, anxiolytics, psychostimulants, and other or unknown substances. What leads to addiction has often hinged on the philosophy of the time.[18] Various models of addiction have been previously postulated by what has been termed the moral model, the cultural model, and the habit model, as well as the disease/genetic model.[19] In the GCC the pendulum appears to swing between the "moral model" and "disease model."[20] This implies that those who have a substance use disorder may be liable for prosecution or labeled as "sick," and therefore treated accordingly. The GCC states are increasingly moving toward a medical approach rather than a judicial one in coming to grips with people with addictions. In Oman, for example, the law explicitly states that drug addicts should seek help from a designated medical setting, but those who are "peddling drugs" would be liable for arrests and incarceration.[21] Elarabi and colleagues have reported that addicts are perceived as the victim of "weakened/breakdown of religiosity."[22] Interestingly, among the general public, addiction was not endorsed as criminal endeavor. Conversely, Al-Subaie and Al-Hajjaj have reported a preference for religious prescriptions for prevention and the treatment of substance use disorder in the Saudi population.[23] In contrast, in a study conducted a decade ago, perhaps representing "bygone generations," Bilal and colleagues examined attitudes toward alcohol and substance misuse, and drugs that cause dependency among residents of the Arab/Muslim population residing in Kuwait ($n = 1,001$) via a Likert-type questionnaire.[24] The majority endorsed a negative view toward substance misuse, and thus harbored a stigma toward those people who are dependent on addictive agents.

From a global perspective, there is an inclination toward legalization; according to the proponents of legalization, the much-heralded "war on drugs" appears to have failed to live up to its aspirations[25]—that is, to eliminate the menace of drug dependency.[26] In a nutshell, the process of drug "liberalization" requires eliminating or reducing the prohibition of mind-altering drugs.[27] In the parlance of the medical approach,

> addiction refers to the harmful or hazardous use of psychoactive substances, including alcohol and illicit drugs. Psychoactive substance use can lead to dependence syndrome—a cluster of behavioral, cognitive, and physiological phenomena that develop after repeated substance use and that typically include a strong desire to take the drug, difficulties in controlling its use, persisting in its use despite harmful consequences, a higher priority given

to drug use than to other activities and obligations, increased tolerance, and sometimes a physical withdrawal state.[28]

Although previously assumed to be a regional or cultural practice, with increased globalization, substance misuse is increasingly recognized to be a global challenge. The emerging data on the magnitude of substance misuse is staggering. Concerning alcohol, its harmful use has been indicated to trigger 3.3 million deaths each year.[29] Some empirical studies have estimated that 15.5 million people qualify to be labeled as having substance use disorders, with a huge concentration of opioid-dependent people.[30] Degenhardt and colleagues have reported that 24.1 million people in the world are psychostimulant dependent.[31] Intravenous drug addiction or illicit drug injection has been reported in all corners of the world, including the GCC.[32] According to the World Health Organization, "injecting drug use is reported in 148 countries, of which 120 have reported the presence of human immunodeficiency virus infection, and acquired immune deficiency syndrome (HIV/AIDS) infection among this population," and the GCC states are no exception.[33] This indicates that substance misuse has more repercussions than simply being about addictive substances. Reflecting the situation in the United Kingdom, Nutt and his colleagues have examined the impact of common substance misuse on the individual and society.[34] Using the technique known as "multiple-criteria decision analysis," alcohol was deemed to be more harmful to society, while heroin, crack cocaine, and methamphetamine (crystal meth) were the most harmful drugs to individuals.

The aim of this chapter is to explore substance abuse in the GCC states. In order to analyze and sufficiently portray the situation in the GCC states, I first explore the extent of drug misuse in the GCC, and, second, survey the available evidence on drug initiation and management in the GCC. Within such an outline, the factors fostering drug initiation and the available services for management of substance use disorders in the GCC are highlighted. The chapter concludes with what could be extrapolated from the present review as final remarks.

THE MAGNITUDE OF SUBSTANCE MISUSE IN THE GULF COOPERATION COUNCIL STATES

Various studies have emerged from the GCC states to indicate the magnitude of substance use disorders.[35] It is worthwhile to note that most of the studies are hospital-based rather than those that are methodologically robust, or community surveys, with a few exceptions.[36] It is also likely that drug dependency, being culturally devalued as a practice, is likely to remain a furtive activity and is therefore inaccessible for researchers. Abou-Saleh, Ghubash, and Daradkeh conducted a survey of substance misuse in Al Ain, a principality of the United Arab Emirates.[37] This study was equipped to solicit tendencies for concealment, if any. These authors first interviewed the male cohort of the study. The survey identified 1 percent of the cohort who "admitted" using illicit drugs. However, when the female counterparts were asked if their male relatives were using illicit drugs, the rate increased to 9 percent.[38] This indicates the high tendency of underreporting when gleaning the rate of drug misuse in the Arab/Islamic community.[39] According to Abou-Saleh, there is "an underreporting of substance misuse by men, which may be related to the stigma of addiction (criminality of illicit drug use and religious prohibition of alcohol use in Muslim communities)."[40]

Al-Haqwi has surveyed the perception of medical trainees in Saudi Arabia, on what the author called "the extent of alcohol and substance abuse in the community."[41] This study unequivocally suggests that these "tomorrow's doctors" perceived that alcohol and substance abuse is a common problem in the community. This seems surprising because ethanol consumption is prohibited in the country. Some of the addictive compounds may exist in the community, even though officially sanctioned as *haram*, meaning that the act is sanctioned as sinful in Islamic jurisprudence.[42] If the condition is ostracized or stigmatized, it becomes a barrier to include it for harm-reduction services.[43] It is also worthwhile to note that certain substances are more available in some regions. For example, due to geography (near the Horn of Africa) and ethnicity, *qat* (*Catha edulis*) is widely used in the Jazan regions of Saudi Arabia.[44] There are also differences in the availability of the context for the use of alcohol.[45] For example, some GCC states (e.g., Bahrain, Qatar, the United Arab Emirates, and Oman) have a relaxed attitude toward marketing alcohol. There is evidence to suggest that alcohol clandestinely enters those states in the GCC with strict alcohol prohibition through smuggling.[46] Zaidan and colleagues have examined the severity of alcohol abuse among Omanis seeking detoxification in one of the tertiary cares in Muscat.[47] They found that the majority of those with a history of alcohol abuse tend to score in the pathological range in the indexes of hazardous and harmful alcohol consumption, the Alcohol Use Disorders Identification Test (called AUDIT). Osman has conducted a retrospective study over a period of one year among patients seeking consultation in a psychiatric hospital in Jeddah.[48] The study found that alcohol was generally consumed at a higher rate of intake compared with other populations. Other studies in the region have alluded to the same view.[49]

Data from the World Health Organization provides some information about alcohol use and the frequency of alcohol use disorders in the GCC states.[50] Based largely on tax data, it is likely that this report underestimates the true consumption of alcohol in the region (table 5.1).

Tobacco is often chewed, sniffed, or smoked either in a cigarette or *shisha*. A *shisha* (also known as a hookah or a hubble bubble) is a smoking device that is widely used on the Arabian Peninsula. Traditionally, both tobacco smoking and its rejuvenated method (waterpipe/*shisha*) are generally condoned,[51] except in Oman.[52] Most smokers consider a *shisha* less harmful to health than cigarette smoking.[53] There is ample evidence to suggest that all forms of ingestion of tobacco have health hazards.[54] In term of its magnitude, Al-Mulla and colleagues conducted a survey investigating the incidence of tobacco consumption among teens (thirteen to fifteen years of age) from the GCC states and Yemen.[55] Their results suggest that these teens have higher rates of tobacco consumption in terms of both *shisha* and cigarettes than their adult counterparts. The "offenders" were teens from Bahrain, Oman, and the United Arab Emirates. The GCC is likely to be experiencing similar encroachment of the tobacco industry, as it has been documented elsewhere in the emerging economy.[56] The situation in the GCC is likely to be ripe for such an undertaking due to the preponderance of the youthful population that often falls prey to the power of tobacco companies marketing within the constraints of existing legislative loopholes.[57]

Many studies have documented the magnitude of polydrug use in the GCC. Data that generalized the situation from North Africa and the Eastern Mediterranean region have estimated that 3,500 per 100,000 of the population of the defined region is dependent on various compounds. The rate of intravenous drug use is 172 per 100,000. The fatalities stemming from drug misuse amount to 9 deaths per 1,000 population. This fatality figure far exceeds the global trend of 4 deaths per 1,000. There are no uniform data to extrapolate the situation meaningfully from that of the GCC. The population of the GCC is unique when compared with North Africa and the Eastern Mediterranean region in many aspects, including economic and social issues, along with those factors that are associated with drug abuse.[58] There are, however, pockets of anecdotal and impressionistic observations on the prevailing trends in the GCC.

Radovanovic and colleagues have screened 3,781 people living in Kuwait.[59] The laboratory analysis indicated that 40 percent of the sample have used hashish, 24 percent were using heroin, and 10 percent were using alcohol.

Table 5.1 **Estimated Gender-Specific Alcohol Use and Alcohol-Associated Disorders in the Gulf Cooperation Council States, 2009**

Country	Alcohol Consumption per Capita (in liters of pure alcohol)		Alcohol Consumption per Capita (Drinkers)[a]		Alcohol Use Disorders (%)[b]	
	Males	*Females*	*Males*	*Females*	*Males*	*Females*
Bahrain	2.7	1.0	23.6	13.9	1.8	0.3
Kuwait	0.2	0.0	0.2	0.0	0.5	0.1
Oman	1.2	0.4	16.5	11.7	0.5	0.1
Qatar	1.8	0.4	24.1	11.1	0.3	0.1
Saudi Arabia	0.3	0.1	4.3	2.7	0.4	0.1
United Arab Emirates	5.5	0.8	34.4	17.8	0.7	0.1

Source: Data from World Health Organization, "Global Status Report on Alcohol and Health," 2014.

[a]Person who consumed at least 60 grams or more of pure alcohol on at least one occasion in the past thirty days.

[b]Based on the scale from the Alcohol Use Disorders Identification Test (AUDIT).

Interestingly, a significant number of those also showed positive for prescription drugs (benzodiazepines and amphetamines.) Jaffer and colleagues conducted a survey examining risk behavior among nationally representative secondary school–based boy and girls in Oman.[60] The study indicates the drug culture is rife; 4.6 percent had consumed tobacco products, 4.3 percent had ingested ethanol, and 4.6 percent admitted to having indulged in illicit drugs. According to Narconon International, a self-proclaimed nonprofit organization that claims to oversee drug rehab and drug education centers around the world,

> Sitting on the Arabian Sea and the Gulf of Oman, not far from the world's largest heroin trafficking channels, . . . Oman was seeing a large increase in the number of those addicted to the drugs. . . . The largest increases in drug addiction are currently seen in school and college girls. In 2008, 1,826 people were officially registered with the government as drug addicts. In 2009, 19 people died due to drug abuse, and the number of crimes related to drug use is escalating, with a rapid increase in the last few years from 78 to 688.[61]

Although the reliability of such figures remains to be established as drug abuse, given that these are furtive activities, such a magnitude could be the tip of the iceberg.[62] Al-Olah and Thiab have reported that approximately 15 percent of admissions to tertiary care in Saudi Arabia were due to drug-related problems.[63] Al Marri and Oei have synthesized the available literature on the type of substances most misused in the GCC.[64] They found that alcohol, heroin, and hashish are the most common types consumed in the GCC. However, this study ostensibly overlooked other types of substances with the potential for misuse, most significantly, prescription medications and volatile solvents.

Most of the quest for establishing the magnitude of substance misuse has been geared toward illicit substances, but there is an increasing recognition that prescription drugs play a significant role in triggering substance misuse disorders. The National Institute on Drug Abuse has classified three classes of prescription drugs that carry a high potential for abuse, including opioids, which are used to treat pain; central nervous system depressants, which are used to treat anxiety and insomnia; and stimulants, which are used as cognitive enhancers, and to induce excessive daytime sleepiness. Little has been foreseen on the prevailing situation of these prescription drugs, with a few exceptions.[65] There is evidence that some emerging chronic conditions are often impervious to available medical treatments. This has led such sufferers to resort to "doctor shopping."[66] Albeit indirectly, this increased prescriptions of medicines that have the potential for addiction.[67] Chronic and refractory conditions, such as haemoglobinopathies, which are widely prevalent in the GCC population, along with the existing laissez-faire attitudes toward the regulation of prescription drugs, could heighten the prevalence of the abuse of prescription drugs.[68]

Although limited to case reports, some studies have indicated the rising tide of the deliberate inhalation of solvents in the GCC.[69] Various terms have been used to describe this type of substance abuse, including volatile substance or toluene abuse. The effect of this type of substance misuse is enormous; the affected individuals tend to develop irreversible and progressive neuro-behavioral impairment.[70] Related to this, there are anecdotal reports of a subculture in the GCC whose members misuse perfume and cologne as intoxicants.[71] Little has been forthcoming in the scholarly literature, but the pattern has been noted in print media, where the tendency to misuse spray deodorants, glue, lighter refills, and spray air fresheners has led to fatal outcomes.[72]

On the whole, though the GCC appears to have a rising tide of substance misuse, some issues have remained conspicuously absent, including the issue of gender. Within the available database, it is difficult to disentangle whether the region follows international trends, or if the situation forms its own unique pattern specific to the GCC. However, there is a strong indication that myriad substances are consumed in the GCC, including alcohol, opiate and opioid analgesics, psycho-stimulants such as *qat*, nonprescribed substances such as amphetamines, prescribed substances, tobacco smoking and its rejuvenated method (waterpipes/*shisha*), and volatile substance abuse.

DRUG INITIATION AND MANAGEMENT IN THE GULF COOPERATION COUNCIL STATES

One crucial question is what fosters the initiation of substance misuse in the GCC. Studies elsewhere have shown that the availability of potential substances for abuse, personality, peer pressure, and the type of the drug consumed all play strong parts in the initiation of drug misuse.[73] Similar precipitating factors appear to exist in the GCC states.[74] Some of these factors are discussed in tandem in the ensuing paragraphs.

First, Oman, the United Arab Emirates, and Bahrain, for example, have clubs where alcohol is readily available to members. In most GCC states, except Saudi Arabia and Kuwait, there are legal outlets for alcoholic beverages. Within such a setting, one can entertain the hypothesis whether availability is a strong predictor of the harmful and hazardous effects of alcohol. Zaidan and colleagues have reported that in Oman there is a strong, direct relationship between availability/accessibility and the resulting alcoholism.[75] If the assumption is that availability has a direct bearing on abuse, then, by definition, most of the substances with potential for dependency in general should not exist in the GCC. With the advent of Islam, the region should have prevailed as free of the malevolence of substance use disorders. This would imply that most of the addictive substances are alien to the region. This means that substances must have clandestinely entered the GCC and are likely to remain in furtive activity.[76] This, in turn, raises concerns; that is, most of the illicit drugs are likely to be found underground, with all the consequences that may ensue in terms of criminal behavior, smuggling, and threats to safety and health.

Second, previous studies of individuals with substance use disorders endorsed the view that boredom was an important precursor of their entry into the world of addiction.[77] This is consistent with the teaching that "an idle mind is the devil's playground." Recent affluence in the region has witnessed increased sedentary life. Lee and colleagues have reported that some GCC nationals are the third most inactive people in the world.[78] On one hand, this has triggered a proliferation of "lifestyle diseases" or "diseases of affluence."[79] On the other hand, the question remains whether a sedentary lifestyle or its extension, boredom, could act as a precursor for some people to use drugs to escape boredom. Studies from other parts of the world do suggest the link between boredom and drug dependency.[80] Because such a link appears rather circuitous, further studies are therefore warranted.

Third, various studies from the GCC have indicated that there is a temporal relationship between underlying temperaments, mental illnesses, and a propensity for the development of substance use disorders.[81] Recent rapid modernization has occurred within the GCC, and youth—who represent an important segment of society—are increasingly experiencing varied acculturations.

Here, it is pertinent to use a model of social behavior developed by Dwairy and Van Sickle to reflect on the prevailing situation in the GCC that could have a direct bearing on drug misuse.[82] This model has three subgroups:

- *People with a traditional cultural identity*, including those who have a strong sense of identification with their own culture and who live according to the traditional norms and values.
- *People with a bicultural, unintegrated identity*, including those who live in the two distinct cultural worlds of Western culture and traditional Arab/Islamic culture. These individuals are essentially culturally split, and might be conceptualized as facing a cultural identity crisis.
- *People with a biculturally well-integrated identity*, including individuals who are able to maintain a harmonious balance of both traditional and Western cultural influences in their personal lives.

Accordingly, in Dwairy and Van Sickle's framework, in addition to the traditional cultural identity represented by those who have a strong sense of identification with typical Arabic/Islamic characteristics, there are also individuals who prescribe to social behaviors that represent society's acculturation and globalization trends, and therefore adhere to social behavior that reflects a bicultural identity. Among those with a bicultural identity, one segment carries an ambivalent affinity for both the traditional value system and the emerging global culture, thus having a split allegiance toward them. There are also a number of youth who have a biculturally well-integrated identity. In their personal lives, such individuals tend to maintain a harmonious balance of both traditional and global cultural influences. Another group consists of those who have totally adopted a Western view of life.[83] A question arises as to which of these social behaviors are likely to succumb to drug addiction. The picture is mixed, given that different types of social behavior have been linked to a propensity for substance misuse.[84] This means that initiations into a drug culture fluctuate in complex ways.

Amir examined the personality profile of heroin, alcohol, and polydrug abusers among what the authors called an "Arabian Gulf population."[85] The study reported that compared with those who do not abuse drugs, individuals with substance use disorders have more characteristics of alienation and unremitting feelings of discomfort. Although a discussion of temperaments has merit, it has been difficult to discern whether an "addictive personality" is a cause or a consequence of substance misuse.[86] In addition to characterological analysis, some studies have alluded to the view that people with substance use disorders have a high propensity to exhibit various psychopathologies. The correlates of substance misuse include a spectrum of various psychiatric conditions.[87] One assumption is that substance misuse is a form of self-medication for existing mental disorders. Another assumption is that the presence of mental disorders in people with substance use disorder is the effect of consuming harmful substances.[88]

In the context of Saudi Arabia, Alsanusy and Setouhy have noted that peer pressure, the desire to show maturity, and ease of availability are some of the factors leading to the initiation of drug dependency.[89] Sheikh and colleagues have examined the quality of life among addicts versus nonaddicts.[90] The study found that addiction is associated with lower educational and social strata. This would imply that education would be one of the channels to combat the vagaries of addiction.

In addition to factors leading to initiation, various studies have explored correlates associated with substance misuse in the GCC. Raheel, Mahmood, and BinSaeed have reported that illicit drug use is strongly associated with premarital sexual activity among defined populations in Riyadh.[91] Here again, this suggests an interesting relationship between drug addiction and other social patterns of behavior.

Njoh and Zimmo have examined the prevalence of HIV/AIDS among attendees with a substance use disorder in Jeddah.[92] The route of heroin administration (parenteral, sharing of needles/syringes) could trigger HIV/AIDS. Among 2,628 screened for HIV, only 4 were confirmed positive. As noted above, intravenous drug use is quite common in the GCC's population. Although the relationship between HIV and intravenous drug use would require further scrutiny in the context of the GCC, the observed low prevalence appears counterintuitive. Data from international trends have indicated a high prevalence of HIV/AIDS among intravenous drug users.[93] Reflecting on the situation, a low prevalence of HIV has appeared in some Islamic countries. The combination of substance use disorder and low HIV/AIDS prevalence has been described as the

"Indian Ocean paradox."[94] There is merit in examining whether such a paradox exists in the GCC.

The last interrelated focus under the umbrella of the pattern and profile of substance misuse is to examine the management of substance use disorders. There are reports that specialized centers for alcohol and drug abuse treatment have cropped up in most of the GCC states. For example, there are eighteen hospitals furnishing the needs of people with substance use disorders. There has also been a growth of private clinics with services relevant for the drug addict population. The existence and development of such private clinics has been a curse in disguise—there are anecdotal reports that these clinics are a veneer for drug peddling and malpractice.[95]

It appears that services for people with substance use disorders are shackled to drug therapy, and the utilization of pharmacological armament often appears to be orthogonal to international best practice.[96] Strict reliance on pharmacological agents is fraught with problems. It has been well established that pharmacological interventions to wean people off drugs are basically limited to mitigating withdrawal symptoms.[97] This implies that nonbiological factors play a significant role in maintaining a compulsion for drug misuse. This will imply that pharmacological treatment is only one part of the answer, as testified by the prevailing situation in the GCC. Some studies have found that relapses are quite common in people with substance use disorder. Rahim and colleagues have indicated that 60 percent of those with substance use disorders tend to relapse in Saudi Arabia, and a similar trend was noted in Kuwait.[98] Iqbal indicated the existence of high dropout rates and low compliance among Saudis with substance use disorders.[99] First, it is possible that substances abused in the GCC might be potent in purer forms, considering that the region is closer to drug-producing countries. Second, Bener and Ghuloum have reported that a significant number of Qataris endorsed the view that psychiatric medication causes addiction (61 percent of attendees in the primary healthcare setting sample).[100] This implies that there is a low threshold of confidence toward biomedical care for substance use disorders. Third, due to genetics, and in combination with sociocultural factors, the GCC's population might have responded differently to those substances of abuse due to differences in pharmacokinetics.[101] This might contribute to the observed high relapse rate in the region.[102]

According to the White House Office of National Drug Control Policy, "treatment of substance use disorder consists of a range of clinical interventions that can include group and individual therapy, medication for detoxification, and stabilization. The ultimate goal of treatment is to assist individuals in achieving stable, long-term recovery, enabling them to become productive, contributing members of society and eliminating the substantial public health, public safety, and economic consequences associated with active addiction."[103] This means safeguarding the well-being of people with substance use disorders is "everybody's business," including those who dispense medical intervention and psychosocial rehabilitation, those who are responsible for providing welfare and harm reduction, and those working in the criminal justice system. Such a comprehensive and multidisciplinary approach has yet to proliferate in the GCC. Most of the discussion concerning the unmet needs of people with substance abuse disorder is a lack of psychosocial intervention.[104] On one hand, most of the widely used psychosocial interventions have yet to be widely introduced into the region. Due to sociocultural teachings, there is some indication that the GCC population is more likely to present their psychosocial needs in a language that is orthogonal to the prescribed in the Euro-American populations. Thus the idiom of distress in the GCC is in the form of somatopsychic rather than psychological, a fear that is consistent with collective sociocultural patterning.[105] This implies that psychosocial rehabilitation would have been a mantled, culturally-sanctioned approach. Many misconstruals in the GCC are often the prerogative of traditional healing systems.[106] The question remains whether the modern healthcare system could adopt some traditional teachings to address some of the unmet psychosocial needs of people with substance use disorder.[107]

CONCLUDING REMARKS

The discourse above has indicated that there are pockets of research in the GCC that address various aspects of substances with the potential for addiction. The available literature is mostly impressionistic, and the bulk of research is skewed toward regional variations.[108] Interestingly, it appears there was a spurt of research output at the turn of the century, but it was then followed by a notable reduction in recent times. It is not clear whether the recent decline in research stems from increased Islamization in the region and if the emergence of narratives that pertain to the region's sociocultural teachings are likely to be unencumbered by the exigencies of the material world, pleasure, and desire.[109] Despite such caveats, the present review suggests that drug dependency is becoming a challenge in the GCC states. Within such a background, the following points are worthwhile to consider if enlightened views toward drug addictions are to be contemplated.

Drawing from the trends presented in the available literature in the GCC, one could easily extrapolate that there is country variation in the magnitude of substance misuse. It appears that those countries adhering to what are meant to be puritanical stances toward addiction tend to incur a higher magnitude of drug dependency, and all the consequences this may entail. But there is a caveat to such a generalization because the opinion here was gauged from the published literature. It is also possible that the "culture of silence" may have led some countries to not publish data on drug addiction. In terms of research on the bibliometrics that are relevant to drug addiction, studies examining opioid abuse in the GCC states have been few and far between.[110] There is also variation in population size among the members of the GCC, which could in turn contribute to variation in the magnitude of drug addictions.

The available services in the GCC have modeled themselves on an Anglo-American model of screening and diagnosis for substance use disorders. Most of the diagnostic tools are gleaned either from the International Classification of Diseases or the *Diagnostic and Statistical Manual of Mental Disorders*.[111] Various studies have emerged from the GCC to testify to this view, and indeed some GCC states do abide by international best practice.[112] Although diagnostic tools should be welcome as a beginning, a conscious effort should be made to make these screening tools relevant to GCC societies. This means that there is a need for standardization of taxonomy relevant to the region. Taxonomic assumptions shape the views of severity of substance use disorder, treatment and administrative decisions, professional communication, formal diagnoses, diagnostic formulations, research, epidemiology, and public policy.

There is a strong indication that due to rudimentary services, the phenomenon of treatment abroad is often the rule rather than the exception for people with substance use disorders.[113] The issue of the treatment approach has the advantage that someone with a substance use disorder will receive treatment from a center with more comprehensive services than those existing in the GCC. This, in turn, reflects upon healthcare services in the GCC, where treatment abroad is much cherished compared with locally available resources. In reference to other types of medical tourism, some drawbacks or unintended consequences are beginning to emerge in the literature.[114] Considering that substance use disorders are refractory conditions, there is little merit to seek a quick fix abroad. The development of local resource is therefore imperative.

In most GCC states, there is an urgent need to address the unmet psychosocial needs of people with substance use disorders. There is a dearth of qualified people to dispense psychosocial interventions. Furthermore, due to differences in sociocultural teachings, there are some indications that treatment methods that are used in other countries may be less effective in the GCC states.[115] Concerted effort is needed to develop and adopt a Western-hybrid model—that is, a blend of Western and GCC-specific approaches. Alternative, indigenous psychosocial interventions also need to be developed. Both these models ought to be evidence based.

It appears opiates and their derivatives are commonly consumed in the GCC on par with patterns observed in other endemic regions, but with some interesting trajectories. In the instance of Oman, among 1,521 people with substance use disorder, 66 percent are intravenous drug abusers.[116] Despite the strong relationship between HIV/AIDS and intravenous drugs in many parts of the world, there is little evidence to suggest that HIV/AIDS is common among drug users in the GCC states.[117] More studies are needed to scrutinize this trend. Similarly, despite the rampant alcoholism that has been reported for the GCC, there is little information on the ill effects of alcoholism in the available literature.

One of the fallouts from drug addiction is the increasing amount of violence and crime. Little has been forthcoming on the relationship between crime and drug misuse in the GCC states. Similarly, there is a dearth of study on drug overdose and drug-related deaths.

According to surveys in the available literature, it appears that dependency of prescription medications is more prevalent in the GCC. This would require a policy to regulate the accessibility of prescription drugs to the public. Most of the countries appear to have failed to abide by international best practice regarding drug control.[118]

Reflecting the situation elsewhere, it is unlikely that the GCC will remain "clean" from the challenges of addiction and its consequences. This means that harm reduction should be prioritized, with an evolving mechanism to liberalize some of the substances that existing science indicates will be less harmful to the individual and society. The pretext that sociocultural teaching will withstand the vagaries of addiction in the GCC states appears to be an untenable aspiration. For example, despite the fact that Ibadhism, the sect of Islam that is predominant in Oman, teaches against smoking, cigarette smoking appears to be rife in Oman.[119] It appears that modern temptations are capable of eroding sociocultural teachings. There has also been a notable erosion of traditional social cohesion, with a marked increase in individualistic persuasion and transformation of the extended family into a nuclear family.[120] The problem of drug abuse is likely to remain acute for the foreseeable future. This partly stems from the preponderance of youth in the GCC population structure, but also from the fact that the region's society is in the midst of a transition from traditional to modern. There are empirical studies indicating that societies in transition tend to be vulnerable to drug abuse, as has been shown in other societies undergoing transition.[121]

Due to the preponderance of youth in the GCC states, concerted efforts are needed to address the needs of this particular portion of the population. Some preliminary studies reveal that drug abuse is trending toward a younger population.[122] In a nutshell, the future and the integrity of the GCC are likely to strongly hinge on how its present opinion leaders fare in safeguarding the well-being of the region's people of tomorrow. More research on this endeavor would likely lead to evidence-based policies and increased allocation of resources.

NOTES

1. A. Al-Harthi and S. Al-Adawi, "Enemy Within? The Silent Epidemic of Substance Dependency in GCC Countries," *Sultan Qaboos University Journal for Scientific Research–Medical Sciences* 4 (2002): 1–7.

2. United Nations Development Program, *Human Development Report 2014: Sustaining Human Progress—Reducing Vulnerabilities and Building Resilience* (New York: United Nations, 2014).

3. L. Al-Lamki, "UN Millennium Development Goals and Oman: Kudos to Oman on Its 40th National Day," *Sultan Qaboos University Medical Journal* 10 (2010): 301–5.

4. M. Barber, M. Mourshed, and F. Whelan, "Improving Education in the Gulf," *McKinsey Quarterly*, 2007, 39–47.

5. T. J. Al-Nasr, "Gulf Cooperation Council (GCC) Women and Misyar Marriage: Evolution and Progress in the Arabian Gulf," *Journal of International Women's Studies* 12, no. 3 (2011): 43–57.

6. S. Zeidan and S. Bahrami, "Women Entrepreneurship in GCC: A Framework to Address Challenges and Promote Participation in a Regional Context," *International Journal of Business and Social Science* 2 (2011): 100–107.

7. International Monetary Fund, "Over 50% of GCC Population under 25," *Middle East Financial News*, July 18, 2012, http://search.proquest.com/docview/1026638215?accountid =27575; D. Tabutin and B. Schoumaker, "The Demography of the Arab World and the Middle East from the 1950s to the 2000s: A Survey of Changes and a Statistical Assessment," *Population* 60 (2005): 505–59.

8. R. Al-Walayti, "The Necessity for Producing Educational Television Programs Nationally in Order to Preserve the National Culture in the Arab States: Case Study of the State of Kuwait" (thesis, University of Massachusetts, Amherst, 1991).

9. "International Conference on Challenges of Urbanization in GCC Countries," Oman News Agency, March 22, 2014, http://search.proquest.com/docview/1509233728?accountid =27575; Ingo Forstenlechner and Emilie Jane Rutledge, "The GCC's 'Demographic Imbalance': Perceptions, Realities and Policy Options," *Middle East Policy* 18 (2011): 25–43.

10. T. A. Al-Barwani and T. S. Albeelyb, "The Omani Family: Strengths and Challenges," *Marriage & Family Review* 41 (2007): 119–42.

11. Reuters, "Immigrant Nannies Worry Persian Gulf," *Los Angeles Times*, October 26, 1986, http://articles.latimes.com/1986-10-26/news/mn-7694_1_foreign-manpower; S. L. Friedman and D. E. Boyle, "Attachment in US Children Experiencing Nonmaternal Care in the Early 1990s," *Attachment and Human Development* 10 (2008): 225–61.

12. Anees Sultan, "A Maid Is Not a Mother, Even if the Children Turn to Her First," *The National*, September 27, 2008, www.thenational.ae/thenationalconversation/comment/a-maid-is-not-a-mother-even-if-the-children-turn-to-her-first.

13. Hamed Al-Sinawi, Mohammed Al-Alawi, Rehab Al-Lawati, Ahmed Al-Harrasi, Mohammed Al-Shafaee, and Samir Al-Adawi, "Emerging Burden of Frail Young and Elderly Persons in Oman: For Whom the Bell Tolls?" *Sultan Qaboos University Medical Journal* 12, no. 2 (2012): 169–76.

14. James McIntosh, Fiona MacDonald, and Neil McKeganey, "The Reasons Why Children in Their Pre- and Early Teenage Years Do or Do Not Use Illegal Drugs," *International Journal of Drug Policy* 16, no. 4 (2005): 254–61.

15. Jack S. Blocker, David M. Fahey, and Ian R. Tyrrell, *Alcohol and Temperance in Modern History: An International Encyclopedia* (Santa Barbara, CA: ABC-CLIO, 2003).

16. American Psychiatric Association, *Diagnostic and Statistical Manual of Mental Disorders: DSM-IV-TR* (Washington, DC: American Psychiatric Publishing, 2000).

17. American Psychiatric Association, *Diagnostic and Statistical Manual of Mental Disorders: DSM-IV-TR* (Washington, DC: American Psychiatric Publishing, 2013).

18. W. A. McKim and S. Hancock, *Drugs & Behavior: Introduction to Behavioral Pharmacology*, 7th ed. (Upper Saddle River, NJ: Pearson, 2012).

19. McKim and Hancock, *Drugs & Behavior*.

20. A. Al Harthi, "Drug Abuse in the Gulf States / Oman: An Evaluation of the Death Penalty as a Deterrent" (thesis, University of Manchester, 1999).

21. Al-Harthi and Al-Adawi, "Enemy Within?"

22. H. Elarabi, F. Al Hamedi, S. Salas, and S. Wanigaratne, "Rapid Analysis of Knowledge, Attitudes and Practices towards Substance Addiction across Different Target Groups in Abu Dhabi City, United Arab Emirates," *International Journal of Prevention and Treatment of Substance Use Disorder* 1 (2013): 76–88.

23. A. S. Al-Subaie and M. S. Al-Hajjaj, "Awareness and Knowledge of Saudi University Students about Drug Dependence," *Saudi Medical Journal* 16 (1995): 326–29.

24. A. M. Bilal, B. Makhawi, G. Al-Fayez, and A. F. Shaltout, "Attitudes of a Sector of the Arab-Muslim Population in Kuwait towards Alcohol and Drug Misuse: An Objective Appraisal," *Drug and Alcohol Dependence* 26 (1990): 55–62.

25. B. Bruce and A. A. Block, "A Trojan Horse: Anti-Communism and the War on Drugs," *Crime, Law and Social Change* 14 (1990): 39–55.

26. Gary Fields, "White House Czar Calls for End to 'War on Drugs,'" *Wall Street Journal*, May 14, 2009, www.wsj.com/articles/SB124225891527617397.

27. W. Hall and J. Lucke, "Drug Decriminalization and Legalization," in *Interventions for Addiction: Comprehensive Addictive Behaviors and Disorders*, ed. Peter M. Miller (New York: Academic Press, 2013), 689–96.

28. World Health Organization, "Substance Abuse," www.who.int/topics/substance_abuse/en/.

29. World Health Organization, "Global Status Report on Alcohol and Health 2014," http://apps.who.int/iris/bitstream/10665/112736/1/9789240692763_eng.pdf.

30. L. Degenhardt, F. Charlson, B. Mathers, W. D. Hall, A. D. Flaxman, N. Johns, and T. Vos, "The Global Epidemiology and Burden of Opioid Dependence: Results from the Global Burden of Disease 2010 Study," *Addiction* 109 (2014): 1320–33.

31. L. Degenhardt, A. J. Baxter, Y. Y. Lee, W. Hall, G. E. Sara, N. Johns, A. Flaxman, H. A. Whiteford, and T. Vos, "The Global Epidemiology and Burden of Psychostimulant Dependence: Findings from the Global Burden of Disease Study 2010," *Drug and Alcohol Dependence* 137 (2014): 36–47.

32. S. Abdel-Baqui, "Personality Characteristics of Heroin Addicted in Saudi Arabia," *Derasat Nafseyah* 2 (1992): 75–101; P. Panduranga, S. Al-Abri, and J. Al-Lawati, "Intravenous Drug Abuse and Tricuspid Valve Endocarditis: Growing Trends in the Middle East Gulf Region," *World Journal of Cardiology* 5 (2013): 397–403.

33. M. K. al-Haddad, A. S. Khashaba, B. Z. Baig, and S. Khalfan, "HIV Antibodies among Intravenous Drug Users in Bahrain," *Journal of Communicable Diseases* 26 (1994): 127–32; J. Njoh and S. Zimmo, "The Prevalence of Human Immunodeficiency Virus among Drug-Dependent Patients in Jeddah, Saudi Arabia," *Journal of Substance Abuse Treatment* 14 (1997): 487–88.

34. D. J. Nutt, L. A. King, and L. D. Phillips, "Drug Harms in the UK: A Multicriteria Decision Analysis," *The Lancet* 376 (2010): 1558–65.

35. Al-Haddad, Khashaba, Baig, and Khalfan, "HIV Antibodies"; S. M. Saleh and A. M. Demerdash, "A Retrospective Study of a Selected Population of Drug Dependent Subjects in Kuwait," *British Journal of Addiction* 73 (1978): 89–92; F. O. El-Anzey and Abel Moneim, "Use of Psychoactive Substances among University Students in Kuwait: An Epidemiological Study," (in Arabic), *Annals of Arts and Social Sciences* 24 (2003): 8–118; F. H. Al-Kandari, K. Yacoub, and F. E. Omu, "Effect of Drug Addiction on the Biopsychosocial Aspects of Persons with Addiction in Kuwait: Nursing Implications," *Journal of Addictions Nursing* 18 (2007): 31–40; M. T. Abou-Saleh, R. Ghubash, and T. Daradkeh, "Al Ain Community Psychiatric Survey I: Prevalence and Socio-Demographic Correlates," *Social Psychiatry and Psychiatric Epidemiology* 36 (2001): 20–28; T. S. AlMarri and T. P. Oei, "Alcohol and Substance Use in the Arabian Gulf Region: A Review," *International Journal of Psychology* 44 (2009): 222–33; Y. O. Younis and A. G. A. Saad, "Profile of Alcohol and Drug Misusers in an Arab Community," *Addiction* 90 (1995): 1683–84; N. A. Qureshi and T. A. Al-Habeeb, "Sociodemographic Parameters and Clinical Pattern of Drug Abuse in Al-Qassim Region—Saudi Arabia," *Arab Journal of Psychiatry* 11 (2000): 10–21; S. Effat, "Patterns of Alcohol and Illicit Drug Use in Kuwait: A Preliminary Study," *New Egyptian Journal of Medicine* 11 (1994): 130–35; A. Okasha, "Young People and the Struggle against Drug Abuse in the Arab Countries," *Bulletin on Narcotics* 37 (1985): 67–73; A. M. Bilal, "Kuwait Drug Addiction Scene: A Changing Pattern?" *International Journal of the Addictions* 24 (1989): 1137–44.

36. Abou-Saleh, Ghubash, and Daradkeh, "Al Ain Community Psychiatric Survey," 20–28.

37. Ibid.

38. Ibid.

39. A. M. Bilal, "Correlates of Addiction-Related Problems in Kuwait: A Cross-Cultural View," *Acta Psychiatrica Scandinavica* 78 (1988): 414–16.

40. M. T. Abou-Saleh, "Substance Use Disorders: Recent Advances in Treatment and Models of Care," *Journal of Psychosomatic Research* 61 (2006): 305–10.

41. Ali I. Al-Haqwi, "Perception among Medical Students in Riyadh, Saudi Arabia, Regarding Alcohol and Substance Abuse in the Community: A Cross-Sectional Survey,"

Substance Abuse Treatment, Prevention, and Policy 5, no. 2 (2010), doi:10.1186/1747-597X
-5-2.

42. A. Northcott, "Substance Abuse," in *Counseling Muslims: Handbook of Mental Health Issues and Interventions*, ed. Sameera Ahmed and Mona M. Amer (New York: Routledge, 2011), 355–82.

43. M. Bassiony, "Substance Use Disorders in Saudi Arabia," *Journal of Substance Use* 18 (2013): 450–66.

44. Kamaludin A. Sheikh, Maged El-setouhy, Umar Yagoud, Rashad Alsanosy, and Zafar Ahmed, "Khat Chewing and Related Quality Of Life: Cross-Sectional Study in Jazan Region, Kingdom of Saudi Arabia," *Health and Quality of Life Outcomes* 12 (2014): 44, doi: 10.1186 /1477-7525-12-44.

45. Ziad Zaidan, Atsu Dorvlo, Nonna Viernes, Abdullah Al-Suleimani, and Samir Al-Adawi, "Hazardous and Harmful Alcohol Consumption among Non-Psychotic Psychiatric Clinic Attendees in Oman," *International Journal of Mental Health and Addiction* 5 (2007): 3–15.

46. Blocker, Fahey, and Tyrrell, *Alcohol and Temperance*.

47. Zaidan et al., "Hazardous and Harmful Alcohol Consumption," 3–15.

48. A. A. Osman, "Substance Abuse among Patients Attending a Psychiatric Hospital in Jeddah: A Descriptive Study," *Annals of Saudi Medicine* 12 (1992): 289–93.

49. A. M. Bilal, E. A. Al-Ansari, J. Kristof, A. Shaltout, and M. F. El-Islam, "Prospective Study of Alcoholism in Kuwait, A 5-Year Follow-Up Report," *Drug and Alcohol Dependence* 23 (1989): 82–86.

50. World Health Organization, "Global Status Report on Alcohol and Health 2014," 2014, http://who.int/substance_abuse/publications/global_alcohol_report/en/.

51. Y. A. Al-Turki, "Smoking Habits among Medical Students in Central Saudi Arabia," *Saudi Medical Journal* 27 (2006), 700–703; S. Al-Bahlani and R. Mabry, "Preventing Non-Communicable Disease in Oman: A Legislative Review," *Health Promotion International* 29, no. S1 (2014): S83–S91, doi: 10.1093/heapro/dau041.

52. Al-Turki, "Smoking Habits," 700–703; Al-Bahlani and Mabry, "Preventing Non-Communicable Disease," S83–S91.

53. S. M. Borgan, G. Jassim, Z. A. Marhoon, M. A. Almuqamam, M. A. Ebrahim, and P. A. Soliman, "Prevalence of Tobacco Smoking among Health-Care Physicians in Bahrain," *BMC Public Health* 14, no. 1 (2014): 931, doi: 10.1186/1471-2458-14-931.

54. S. F. Al-Fayez, M. Salleh, M. Ardawi, and F. M. Zahran, "Effects of Sheesha and Cigarette Smoking on Pulmonary Function of Saudi Males and Females," *Tropical and Geographical Medicine* 40 (1988): 115–23; K. Al-Umran, O. M. Mahgoub, and N.Y. Qurashi, "Volatile Substance Abuse among School Students of Eastern Saudi Arabia," *Annals of Saudi Medicine* 13 (1993): 520–24; S. F. Al-Fayez, M. Ardawi, and F. M. Zahran, "Carboxyhemoglobin Concentrations in Smokers of Sheesha and Cigarettes in Saudi Arabia," *British Medical Journal* (Clinical Research Education) 291 (1985): 1768–70; W. Maziak, K. D. Ward, R. A. Soweid, and T. Eissenberg, "Tobacco Smoking Using a Waterpipe: A Re-Emerging Strain in a Global Epidemic," *Tobacco Control* 13 (2004): 327–33.

55. A. Moh'd Al-Mulla, S. Abdou Helmy, J. Al-Lawati, S. Al Nasser, S. Ali Abdel Rahman, A. Almutawa, B. Abi Saab, A. M. Al-Bedah, A. M. Al-Rabeah, A. Ali Bahaj, F. El-Awa, C. W. Warren, N. R. Jones, and S. Asma, "Prevalence of Tobacco Use among Students Aged 13–15 Years in Health Ministers' Council / Gulf Cooperation Council Member States, 2001–2004," *Journal of School Health* 78 (2008): 337–43.

56. Al-Mulla et al., "Prevalence of Tobacco Use," 337–43.

57. O. A. Al-Mohrej, S. I. AlTraif, H. M. Tamim, and H. Fakhoury, "Will Any Future Increase in Cigarette Price Reduce Smoking in Saudi Arabia?" *Annals of Thoracic Medicine* 9 (2014): 154–57; L. Joossens and M. Raw, "From Cigarette Smuggling to Illicit Tobacco Trade," *Tobacco Control* 21 (2012): 230–34.

58. Z. Alam Mehrjerdi, R. Noori, and K. Dolan, "Opioid Use, Treatment and Harm Reduction Services: The First Report from the Persian Gulf Region," *Journal of Substance Misuse* (2014): 1–7, doi:10.3109/14659891.2014.966344.

59. Z. Radovanovic, C. W. Pilcher, T. al-Nakib, and A. Shihab-Eldeen, "On Substance Abuse in Kuwait (1992–1997): Evidence from Toxicological Screening of Patients," *Journal of Substance Abuse* 12 (2000): 363–71.

60. Y. A. Jaffer, M. Afifi, F. Al Ajmi, and K. Alouhaishi, "Knowledge, Attitudes and Practices of Secondary-School Pupils in Oman I: Health-Compromising Behaviour," *Mediterranean Health Journal* 12 (2006): 35–49.

61. Narconon International, "Oman Drug Addiction," *Narconon International*, www.narconon.org/drug-information/oman-drug-addiction.html.

62. Panduranga, Al-Abri, and Al-Lawati, "Intravenous Drug Abuse."

63. Y. H. Al-Olah and K. M. A. Thiab, "Admissions through the Emergency Department Due to Drug-Related Problems," *Annals of Saudi Medicine* 28 (2008): 426–29.

64. AlMarri and Oei, "Alcohol and Substance Use."

65. M. A. Zahid, A. M. Al-Fekki, H. Abdul-Einin, H. Badr, and A. A. Shahid, "Amineptine Abuse: A Study of 203 Patients Abusing Amineptine," *International Journal of Mental Health and Addiction* 7 (November 2004), www.ecommunity-journal.com/pdf/c01a17.pdf; N. Iqbal, "Recoverable Hearing Loss with Amphetamines and Other Drugs," *Journal of Psychoactive Drugs* 36 (2003): 285–88.

66. Al-Sinawi et al., "Emerging Burden."

67. Ola Salem, "Psychiatrists in GCC Blacklisted for Prescribing Drugs Leading to Addiction," *The National*, February 3, 2014, www.thenational.ae/uae/health/psychiatrists-in-gcc-blacklisted-for-prescribing-drugs-leading-to-addiction#ixzz3G2y10oMg.

68. H. A. Hamamy and N. A. Al-Allawi, "Epidemiological Profile of Common Haemoglobinopathies in Arab Countries," *Journal of Community Genetics* 4 (2013): 147–67; J. Elander, J. Lusher, D. Bevan, and P. Telfer, "Pain Management and Symptoms of Substance Dependence among Patients with Sickle Cell Disease," *Social Science & Medicine* 57 (2003): 1683–96.

69. Al-Umran, Mahgoub, and Qurashi, "Volatile Substance Abuse"; R. K. Gupta, J. Van Der Meulen, and K.V. Johny, "Oliguric Acute Renal Failure due to Glue-Sniffing: Case Report," *Scandinavian Journal of Urology* 25 (1991): 247–50; A. S. Omar, M. U. Rahman, and S. Abuhasna, "Reported Survival with Severe Mixed Acidosis and Hyperlactemia after Toluene Poisoning," *Saudi Journal of Anaesthesia* 5 (2011): 73–75; D. Deleu and Y. Hanssens, "Cerebellar Dysfunction in Chronic Toluene Abuse: Beneficial Response to Amantadine Hydrochloride," *Journal of Clinical Toxicology* 38 (2000): 37–41.

70. C. M. Filley, "Toluene Abuse and White Matter: A Model of Toxic Leukoencephalopathy," *Psychiatric Clinics of North America* 36 (2013): 293–302.

71. Raynald C. Rivera, "New 'Regulations Won't Hit Perfume Industry,'" *The Peninsula*, February 7, 2013, http://search.proquest.com/docview/1370961467?accountid=27575.

72. "Saudi Arabia: 19 Die after Drinking Cologne Laced with Methanol," *National Post*, June 11, 2002, http://search.proquest.com/docview/330066363?accountid=27575.

73. C. L. Storr, F. A. Wagner, C. Y. Chen, and J. C. Anthony, "Childhood Predictors of First Chance to Use and Use of Cannabis by Young Adulthood," *Drug and Alcohol Dependence* 117 (2011): 7–15.

74. Al-Kandari, Yacoub, and Omu, "Effect of Drug Addiction"; N. al-Nahedh, "Relapse among Substance-Abuse Patients in Riyadh, Saudi Arabia," *Eastern Mediterranean Health Journal* 5 (1999): 241–46; N. Iqbal, "Substance Dependence: A Hospital-Based Survey," *Saudi Medical Journal* 21 (2000): 51–57; A. M. Bilal and M. Angelo-Khattar, "Correlates of Alcohol-Related Causality in Kuwait," *Acta Psychiatrica Scandinavica* 78 (1988): 417–20.

75. Zaidan et al., "Hazardous and Harmful Alcohol Consumption."

76. Blocker, Fahey, and Tyrrell, "Alcohol and Temperance."

77. Al-Harthi, "Drug Abuse."

78. I. M. Lee, E. J. Shiroma, F. Lobelo, P. Puska, S. N. Blair and P. T. Katzmarzyk, "Effect of Physical Inactivity on Major Non-Communicable Diseases Worldwide: An Analysis of Burden of Disease and Life Expectancy," *The Lancet* 380 (2012): 219–29.

79. S. Al-Adawi, "Emergence of Diseases of Affluence in Oman: Where Do They Feature in the Health Research Agenda?" *Sultan Qaboos University Medical Journal* 6 (2006): 3–9.

80. A. Rahman, "Drug Addiction: A Pilot Study in Dhaka City," *Personality and Individual Differences* 13 (1992): 119–21; S. J. MacLean, J. Kutin, D. Best, A. Bruun, and R. Green, "Risk Profiles for Early Adolescents Who Regularly Use Alcohol and Other Drugs Compared with Older Youth," *Vulnerable Children and Youth Studies* 9 (2014): 17–27.

81. T. Amir, "Personality Study of Alcohol, Heroin, and Polydrug Abusers in an Arabian Gulf Population," *Psychological Reports* 74 (1994): 515–20; M. Abu-Arab and E. Hashem, "Some Personality Correlates in a Group of Drug Addicts," *Personality and Individual Differences* 19 (1995): 649–53; R. R. Chinnian, L. R. Taylor, A. Al Subaie, A. Sugumar, and A. A. Al Jumaih, "A Controlled Study of Personality Patterns in Alcohol and Heroin Abusers in Saudi Arabia," *Journal of Psychoactive Drugs* 26 (1994): 85–88; T. Amir, "Comparison of Patterns of Substance Abuse in Saudi Arabia and the United Arab Emirates," *Social Behavior and Personality* 29 (2001): 519–30.

82. M. Dwairy and T. D. Van Sickle, "Western Psychotherapy in Traditional Arabic Societies," *Clinical Psychology Review* 16 (1996): 231–49.

83. S. Al-Adawi, "Adolescence in Oman," in *International Encyclopedia of Adolescence: A Historical and Cultural Survey of Young People around the World*, ed. Jeffrey Jensen Arnett (New York: Routledge, 2006), 713–28.

84. A. S. Al-Subaie and M. S. Al-Hajjaj, "Awareness and Knowledge of Saudi University Students about Drug Dependence," *Saudi Medical Journal* 16 (1995): 326–29; Sheikh et al., "Khat Chewing"; A. A. Yousef, "Drug Problem and Social Change in Saudi Arabia: A Study of the Attitude of Saudi Students Studying in the United States of America towards Drug Use in Saudi Arabia" (thesis, Western Michigan University, 1991); H. Y. Al-Kendary, "Factors of Recidivism among Relapsed and Recovered Drug Addicts in Kuwaiti Society," *Journal of the Social Sciences* 42 (2014): 11–47; R. M. Alsanosy, M. S. Mahfouz, and A. M. Gaffar, "Khat Chewing among Students of Higher Education in Jazan region, Saudi Arabia: Prevalence, Pattern, and Related Factors," BioMed Research International, 2013, doi:10.1155/2013 /487232; F. Daradkeh and H. F. Moselhy, "Death Anxiety (Thanatophobia) among Drug Dependents in an Arabic Psychiatric Hospital," *American Journal of Drug and Alcohol Abuse* 37 (2011): 184–88.

85. Amir, "Personality Study."

86. Abdel-Baqui, "Personality Characteristics"; A. M. Demerdash, H. Mizaal, S. E. El

Farouki, and H. Mossalem, "Some Behavioural and Psychosocial Aspects of Alcohol and Drug Dependence in Kuwait Psychiatric Hospital," *Acta Psychiatrica Scandinavica* 63 (1981): 173–85.

87. Al-Sinawi et al., "Emerging Burden"; R. A. Suleiman, A. S. Khashaba, and M. K. Al-Haddad, "Depressive Symptoms among HIV Positive Drug Users in Bahrain," *Arab Journal of Psychiatry* 13 (2002): 31–35; N. A. Qureshi, "Sociodemographic Correlates, Pattern and Comorbidity of Drug Abuse among Psychiatric Patients," *Arab Journal of Psychiatry* 2 (1992): 98–106; A. M. Bilal and M. F. El-Islam, "Some Clinical and Behavioural Aspects of Patients with Alcohol Dependence Problems in Kuwait Psychiatric Hospital," *Alcohol and Alcoholism* 20 (1985): 57–62.

88. Al-Harthi and Al-Adawi, "Enemy Within?"

89. R. Alsanusy and M. El-Setouhy, "Why Would Khat Chewers Quit? An In-Depth, Qualitative Study on Saudi Khat Quitters," *Substance Abuse* 34 (2013): 389–95.

90. Sheikh et al., "Khat Chewing."

91. H. Raheel, M. A. Mahmood, and A. BinSaeed, "Sexual Practices of Young Educated Men: Implications for Further Research and Health Education in the Kingdom of Saudi Arabia," *Oxford Journal of Public Health* 35 (2013): 21–26.

92. Njoh and Zimmo, "Prevalence of Human Immunodeficiency Virus."

93. C. Aceijas, G. V. Stimson, M. Hickman, and T. Rhodes, "Global Overview of Injecting Drug Use and HIV Infection among Injecting Drug Users," *AIDS* 18 (2004): 2295–303.

94. Y. Dada, F. Milord, E. Frost, J. P. Manshande, A. Kamuragiye, J. Youssouf, M. Khelifa, and J. Pépin, "The Indian Ocean Paradox Revisited: HIV and Sexually Transmitted Infections in the Comoros," *International Journal of STD & AIDS* 18 (2007): 596–600.

95. Salem, "Psychiatrists in GCC Blacklisted"; Y. Amin, E. Hamdi, and R. Ghubash, "Substance Abuse Consultation Rates: Experience from Private Practice in Dubai," *Arab Journal of Psychiatry* 7 (1996): 133–39.

96. A. M. Bilal, J. Kristof, A. Shaltout, and M. F. El-Islam, "Treatment of Alcoholism in Kuwait: A Prospective Follow-Up Study," *Drug and Alcohol Dependence* 19 (1987): 131–44; F. A. Al-Delaim, "Management of Substance Abuse in Saudi Arabia," *Derasat Nafseyah* 7 (1997): 470–84; M. Abdel-Mawgoud and M. K. Al-Haddad, "Heroin Addiction in Bahrain: 15 Years Experience," *Addiction* 91 (1996): 1859–64; B. A. Abalkhail, "Social Status, Health Status and Therapy Response in Heroin Addicts," *Eastern Mediterranean Health Journal* 7 (2001): 465–72; H. V. Hogerzeil, J. Liberman, V. J. Wirtz, S. P. Kishore, S. Selvaraj, R. Kiddell-Monroe, F. N. Mwangi-Powell, and T. von Schoen-Angerer, "Promotion of Access to Essential Medicines for Non-Communicable Diseases: Practical Implications of the UN Political Declaration," *The Lancet* 381 (2013): 680–89; A. M. Kaki, M. F. Daghistani, and A. A. Msabeh, "Nurses' Knowledge of Pharmacological Measures on Acute Pain Management in Western Saudi Arabia," *Saudi Medical Journal* 30 (2009): 279–83.

97. Al-Harthi and Al-Adawi, "Enemy Within?"

98. Al-Nahedh, "Relapse"; E. S. S. El Geili and T. Z. Bashir, "Precipitants of Relapse among Heroin Addicts," *Addictive Disorders and Their Treatment* 4 (2005): 29–38; S. I. A. Rahim, M. S. Abumadani, M. S. Khalil, and T. Musa, "Long-Term Outcome of Treated Addiction in Saudi Arabia: Predictors of Relapse in 10-Year-Follow-Up," *Arab Journal of Psychiatry* 16 (2005): 86–97; Al-Kendary, "Factors of Recidivism."

99. N. Iqbal, "Problems with Inpatient Drug Users in Jeddah," *Annals of Saudi Medicine* 21 (2001): 196–200.

100. A. Bener and S. Ghuloum, "Ethnic Differences in the Knowledge, Attitude and Beliefs towards Mental Illness in a Traditional Fast-Developing Country," *Psychiatria Danubina* 23 (2011): 157–64.

101. Lionel D. Edwards, J. M. Husson, E. Labbé, C. Naito, M. P. Amati, S. Walker, R. L. Williams, and H. Yasurhara, "Racial and Ethnic Issues in Drug Regulation," in *Principles and Practice of Pharmaceutical Medicine*, 3rd ed., ed. Lionel D. Edwards, Anthony W. Fox, and Peter D. Stonier (London: Wiley-Blackwell, 2010), 233–49; K. M. Lin, D. Anderson, and R. E. Poland, "Ethnicity and Psychopharmacology: Bridging the Gap," *Psychiatric Clinics of North America* 18 (1995): 635–47.

102. Rahim et al., "Long-Term Outcome."

103. White House Office of National Drug Control Policy, www.whitehouse.gov/ondcp/about.

104. V. Curran and C. Drummond, "Psychological Treatment of Substance Misuse and Dependence," *Foresight Brain Science: Addiction and Drugs Project*, Office of Science and Technology, UK Department of Trade and Industry, 2005, www.foresight.gov.uk/Brain_Science_Addiction_and_Drugs/Reports_and_Publications/ ScienceReviews/Psychological%20Treatments.pdf.

105. S. Dilworth, I. Higgins, V. Parker, B. Kelly, and J. Turner, "Patient and Health Professional's Perceived Barriers to the Delivery of Psychosocial Care to Adults with Cancer: A Systematic Review," *Psychoencology* 23 (2014): 601–12.

106. S. Al-Adawi, A. Salmi, R. G. Martin, and H. Ghassani, "Zar: Group Distress and Healing," *Mental Health, Religion and Culture* 4 (2001): 47–61

107. S. Tahhoub-Schulte, A. Y. Ali, and T. Khafaji, "Treating Substance Dependency in the UAE: A Case Study," *Journal of Muslim Mental Health* 4 (2009): 67–75.

108. Z. Alam Mehrjerdi, R. Noori, and K. Dolan, "Opioid Use, Treatment and Harm Reduction Services: The First Report from the Persian Gulf Region, *Journal of Substance Misuse*, 2014, 1–7, doi: 10.3109/14659891.2014.966344.

109. A. Torab, "Women and Islamization: Contemporary Dimensions of Discourse on Gender Relations," *American Ethnologist* 27 (2000): 1005–6.

110. Alam Mehrjerdi, Noori, and Dolan, "Opioid Use."

111. World Health Organization, *The ICD-10 Classification of Mental and Behavioural Disorders: Clinical Descriptions and Diagnostic Guidelines* (Geneva: World Health Organization, 1992); American Psychiatric Association, *Diagnostic and Statistical Manual of Mental Disorders* (Washington, DC: American Psychiatric Association, 2000).

112. A. M. Bilal, J. Kristof, and M. F. El-Islam, "A Cross-Cultural Application of a Drinking Behaviour Questionnaire," *Addictive Behaviors* 12 (1987): 95–101; E. A. Al-Ansari and J. C. Negrete, "Screening for Alcoholism among Alcohol Users in a Traditional Arab Muslim Society," *Acta Psychiatrica Scandinavica* 81 (1990): 284–88; T. S. AlMarri, T. P. Oei, and T. Amir, "Validation of the Alcohol Use Identification Test in a Prison Sample Living in the Arabian Gulf Region," *Substance Use & Misuse* 44 (2009): 2001–213; A. M. Bilal, M. A. Khattar, K. I. Hassan, and D. Berry, "Psychosocial and Toxicological Profile of Drug Misuse in Male Army Conscripts in Kuwait," *Acta Psychiatrica Scandinavica* 86 (1992): 104–7; T. S. AlMarri, T. P. Oei, and R. M. Abulrahman, "Validation of the Drinking Refusal Self-Efficacy Questionnaire in Arab and Asian Samples," *Addictive Behaviors* 34 (2009): 776–78; A. Albrithen, "Measuring Alcohol Craving in Saudi Arabia with Possible Implications for Social Work Intervention," *International Journal of Social Welfare* 22 (2013): 384–95; Hogerzeil et al., "Promotion of Access to Essential Medicines."

113. Noimot Olayiwola, "Up to 5% of Population Addicted to Alcohol or Drugs," *Gulf Times*, April 29, 2013, www.gulf-times.com/Mobile/Qatar/178/details/350808/%E2%80%98Up-to-5%25-of-population%E2%80%99-addicted-to-alcohol-or-drugs.

114. J. A. Al-Khalidi, B. Alenezi, W. Al-Qabandy, E. Abo-Hamra, K. Husain, H. A. Askar,

A. P. Jagannathan, H. Abu-El-Naga, and G. W. Neff, "Complications in Paediatric Liver Transplant from Kuwait When Transplanted Abroad," *Arab Journal of Gastroenterology* 13 (2012): 178–79; A. Whittaker and H. L. Chee, "Perceptions of an 'International Hospital' in Thailand by Medical Travel Patients: Cross-Cultural Tensions in a Transnational Space," *Social Sciences & Medicine* 124 (2014): 290–97, doi:10.1016/j.socscimed.2014.10.002.

115. Dwairy and Van Sickle, "Western Psychotherapy."

116. Panduranga, Al-Abri, and Al-Lawati, "Intravenous Drug Abuse."

117. Al-Haddad et al., "HIV Antibodies"; Njoh and Zimmo, "Prevalence of Human Immunodeficiency Virus."

118. Hogerzeil et al., "Promotion of Access to Essential Medicines."

119. A. A. Al Riyami and M. Afifi, "Smoking in Oman: Prevalence and Characteristics of Smokers," *Eastern Mediterranean Health Journal* 10 (2004): 600–609.

120. T. J. Al-Nasr, "Gulf Cooperation Council (GCC) Women and Misyar Marriage: Evolution and Progress in the Arabian Gulf," *Journal of International Women's Studies* 12, no. 3 (2011): 43–57.

121. T. Elton-Marshall, S. T. Leatherdale, and R. Burkhalter, "Tobacco, Alcohol and Illicit Drug Use among Aboriginal Youth Living Off-Reserve: Results from the Youth Smoking Survey," *Canadian Medical Association Journal* 183, no. 8 (2011): 480–648.

122. K. Chaleby, "A Comparative Study of Alcoholics and Drug Addicts in an Arabian Gulf Country," *Social Psychiatry* 21 (1986): 49–51.

A CHRONIC DISEASE PROFILE OF THE GULF COOPERATION COUNCIL STATES

Cother Hajat

In all the Gulf Cooperation Council (GCC) states, there has been an un-precedented increase in wealth and modernization. This, together with an increasingly aging population, has manifested in a dramatic shift in lifestyle and lifestyle-related chronic diseases. These behavioral factors—which include dietary patterns, physical inactivity, and tobacco smoking—have resulted in rapid increases in the prevalence of the risk factors of chronic disease.

Large, population-based prevalence studies are sparse in the research-poor GCC region. One of the most comprehensive reviews of the health status of the Arab population utilizes data from the GBD (Global Burden of Disease) project, which provides modeled estimates of risk factors, morbidity, and mortality.[1] The report demonstrated that though the disease burden in the whole Arab world decreased from 1990 to 2010, the combined morbidity and mortality burden from noncommunicable diseases had increased during this period. Ischaemic heart disease; mental disorders, such as depression and anxiety; musculoskeletal disorders, including lower back pain and neck pain; diabetes; and cirrhosis formed a large proportion of the disease burden of the Arab world in 2010.[2]

In the review, chronic diseases and road injuries were the leading causes of death in the GCC member states and other high-income countries. Road injuries and major depressive disorder were the top two causes of disability-adjusted life-years (known as DALYs), which take into account both mortality and morbidity, whereas cardiovascular disease (CVD) burden was highest in the age group fifty to fifty-nine years. With regard to risk factors, dietary factors were the leading risk for death in all high-income countries, with the exception of Saudi Arabia, where high blood pressure ranked higher. Ischaemic heart disease and CVD were the first and second causes of death in Kuwait and Saudi Arabia. Chronic kidney disease was the sixth commonest cause of death in Oman, Saudi Arabia, and Bahrain; eighth in Kuwait; and ninth in Qatar. In 2010 motor vehicle collisions caused the greatest number of deaths in Qatar, were the second-highest cause of death in the United Arab Emirates and Oman, and the third-highest in Saudi Arabia, Bahrain, and Kuwait.

Although the data provided by the GBD study are very informative, the abundant data in the region are otherwise scarcely reported to provide a status of health outcomes of the GCC, with the majority of articles describing the Middle East Burden of Health. Due to the diversity of ancestry, history, environment, culture, and lifestyles—together with the range of low-, low-middle-, middle-, and high-income countries in the Middle East region—the data do not sufficiently describe the state of health for the GCC states, which all fall into the high-income category.

This chapter aims to quantify the chronic disease burden of the GCC states individually and as a region, and to compare this against suitable benchmark countries. There are numerous tools to monitor the performance of healthcare systems, ranging from self-perceived health status, to measured health status, to the quality of healthcare delivery. The Organization for Economic Cooperation and Development's (OECDs) 2011 framework health indicators, "Health at a Glance, 2011," were chosen due to the availability of data for these measures; the close fit of these data with the known and perceived health burdens in the GCC; and the ability to compare the findings with reliable benchmark data from the OECD member countries.[3]

DATA

The OECD's publication presents data for all its (then) thirty-four member countries, including four new members: Chile, Estonia, Israel, and Slovenia (Latvia has since joined, in 2016). Where possible, it also reports comparable data for Brazil, China, India, Indonesia, the Russian Federation, and South Africa, as major non-OECD economies.[4]

Data for the GCC states were sourced from publicly available data using the World Health Organization's (WHO) global data repositories and local data repositories such as the health authorities, statistics centers, universities, surveys, and other sources. All the data included in this report were representative of all the nationalities living in the GCC states and were not restricted to the nationals only. The following indicators from the OECD domains were reported on:

Health status:
- CVD mortality
- Cancer mortality
- Diabetes prevalence rate

Nonmedical determinants of health:
- Tobacco consumption
- Obesity in adults

Data for the year closest to the data from the OECD indicator were sourced and used only if within two years of the OECD date. The data were reported in the same units as the OECD framework and were plotted in the same format as the OECD graphs.[5] Those OECD framework indicators for which data were not available for all the GCC states were omitted.

FINDINGS

This section presents results for risk factors and health status related to chronic disease in the GCC states. Risk factors are useful predictors of future health status—for example, in disease projections—and changes over time are likely to be reflected earlier in risk factor prevalence rates than in changes of health status.

Risk Factors

Risk factors for chronic disease are a valuable measure of the health status and future health expenditures of a nation.

OBESITY

Obesity is a measure now widely used globally due to its consistent increase in low-, middle-, and high-income settings. The data show that the rates of obesity are at the highest end of the spectrum, alongside those of the United States, for all the GCC states except Oman, where obesity rates in younger age groups are already high, which will eventually lead to increases in the adult population.[6] The rates were highest in Kuwait, at 43 percent; and the other GCC states were fairly similar, at 33 to 35 percent. These data are not age-standardized; after age-standardization, rates of obesity in all GCC states are likely to exceed those of the United States, due to the much younger age of the GCC population. Oman is the exception, with a rate similar to the OECD mean, at 22 percent (fig. 6.1).

DIABETES PREVALENCE

The prevalence of diabetes in all GCC states exceeds rates of the comparison countries, at 12 to 22 percent of the population. The rate is highest in Saudi Arabia, at 22 percent, and lowest in Qatar and Oman, at 12 percent (fig. 6.2).

TOBACCO SMOKING RATES

Tobacco smoking rates in the GCC states are variable. The highest rates are seen in Kuwait at 24 percent, and Saudi Arabia at 22 percent, similar to the OECD average. The rates in other GCC states are relatively low, with 11 percent in the United Arab Emirates and the lowest rate of all countries in Oman, at 7 percent (fig. 6.3).

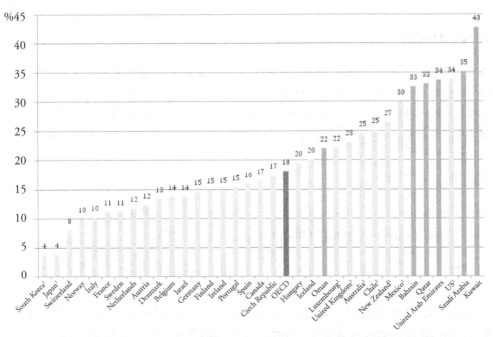

Figure 6.1   **Prevalence Rates for Obesity among the Adult Population in the GCC States in Comparison with the Countries That Belong to the Organization for Economic Cooperation and Development, 2009 (or nearest year)**

Source: Data from World Obesity Federation, "World Map of Obesity," www.world obesity.org/aboutobesity/world-map-obesity/.

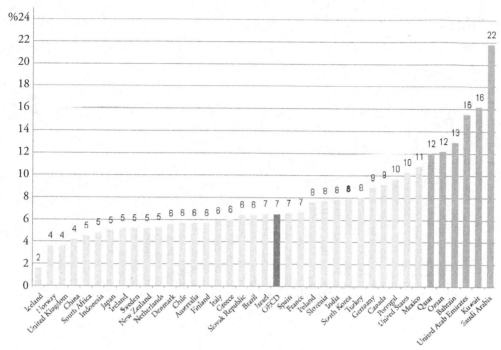

Figure 6.2   **Prevalence Rate for Diabetes Mellitus in the GCC States in Comparison with Other Countries, 2010 (or nearest year)**

Source: Data from World Health Organization, "United Arab Emirates Statistics Summary (2002–present)," http://apps.who.int/ghodata/?vid=20500&theme=country#.

Note: The data cover both Type 1 and Type 2 diabetes. Data are age-standardized to the World Standard Population.

Health Status

The measures of health status include mortality for CVD and cancer. These are briefly examined here.

CARDIOVASCULAR DISEASE MORTALITY

The age-standardized mortality rate for CVD in the GCC states is variable, with Qatar and Bahrain demonstrating rates similar to the OECD average, at 157 and 187 per 100,000 population (fig. 6.4).

CANCER MORTALITY

The age-standardized mortality for cancer, by contrast, is strikingly lower in all the GCC states compared with the OECD countries, at 63 to 101 per 100,000 population, which is less than half the average (fig. 6.5).

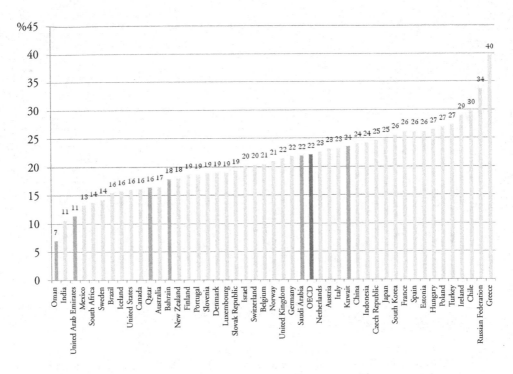

Figure 6.3 **Prevalence Rates for Tobacco Smoking in the GCC States in Comparison with the Countries That Belong to the Organization for Economic Cooperation and Development and Russia**

Source: Data from "OECD Health Data 2007: Statistics and Indicators for 30 Countries," 2007, www.oecd.org/els/health-systems/health-data.htm.

DISCUSSION

This chapter presents a comprehensive comparison of the chronic disease health status of the GCC states with each other and with OECD countries and elsewhere. The comparison shows that, overall, there is a very high burden of CVD, and its risk factors in all GCC states far exceeds that of the OECD comparison countries. Oman is the exception, with a burden more similar to the OECD average. In contrast, cancer mortality rates for all the GCC states were lower than comparison countries, with rates less than half the OECD average (the possible reasons for this are discussed below). There is considerable variation between the GCC states, with Oman and Bahrain demonstrating the lowest burden, and Saudi Arabia and the United Arab Emirates the highest burden. Diabetes mellitus and obesity rates show extremes of prevalence for the GCC states, but tobacco smoking rates are lower than in most comparison countries.

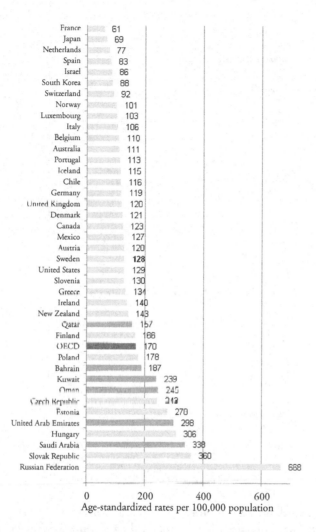

France | 61
Japan | 69
Netherlands | 77
Spain | 83
Israel | 86
South Korea | 88
Switzerland | 92
Norway | 101
Luxembourg | 103
Italy | 106
Belgium | 110
Australia | 111
Portugal | 113
Iceland | 115
Chile | 116
Germany | 119
United Kingdom | 120
Denmark | 121
Canada | 123
Mexico | 127
Austria | 120
Sweden | **128**
United States | 129
Slovenia | 130
Greece | 134
Ireland | 140
New Zealand | 148
Qatar | 157
Finland | 166
OECD | 170
Poland | 178
Bahrain | 187
Kuwait | 239
Oman | 245
Czech Republic | 242
Estonia | 270
United Arab Emirates | 298
Hungary | 306
Saudi Arabia | 338
Slovak Republic | 360
Russian Federation | 668

0   200   400   600
Age-standardized rates per 100,000 population

Figure 6.4   **Age-Standardized Mortality Rate for Cardiovascular Disease in the GCC States in Comparison with the Countries That Belong to the Organization for Economic Cooperation and Development and Russia**

Source: Data from "OECD Health Data 2007: Statistics and Indicators for 30 Countries," 2007, www.oecd.org/els/health-systems/health-data.htm.

RISK FACTORS FOR CHRONIC DISEASE

Risk factors that are influenced by lifestyle changes such as obesity and diabetes are markedly high in the whole GCC region. In the *International Diabetes Federation Atlas, 5th Edition*, six of the top ten prevalence rates for diabetes were in the GCC region.[7] Although there is wide variation in diabetes rates between the GCC states, all are higher than the comparison countries.

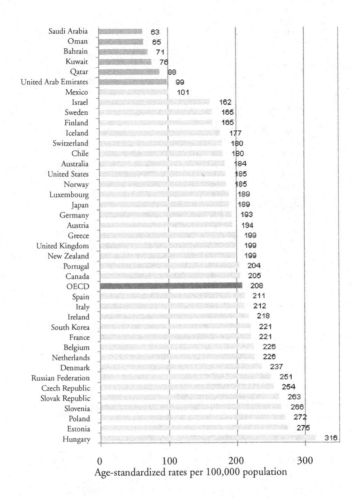

Figure 6.5   **Age-Standardized Mortality Rate for All Cancers in the GCC States in Comparison with the Countries That Belong to the Organization for Economic Cooperation and Development and Russia**

Source: Data from www.oecd.org/els/health-systems/health-data.htm.

The WHO published a set of voluntary global 2025 targets for the prevention and control of noncommunicable diseases as part of its Global Monitoring Framework.[8] The Global Monitoring Target is a halt in the rise in diabetes by 2025. However, without the presence of passive data-collection systems such as diabetes registries, the detection of changes in rates relies on active data collection and may be subject to error. Specific interventions for the prevention of diabetes have not been tested in the GCC and should be considered a priority—

for example, to prevent progression from pre-diabetes to diabetes. The long-term cost-effectiveness of screening for diabetes in the high-prevalence GCC states is unknown. However, there is sufficient evidence to justify the benefit of screening in young adults to avoid the cost and complications of undetected diabetes. With the uniformly high rates of diabetes and pre-diabetes in young populations seen in the GCC states, screening should be an inherent part of the healthcare delivery system. The early detection of diabetes and pre-diabetes through screening will lead to lower costs of care for diabetes, which already accounts for a large proportion of the total healthcare budget in the GCC states, as suggested by local studies on the cost of diabetes care with and without screening and complications.[9]

Obesity rates for most of the GCC states also fall within the top ten rates globally.[10] In order to meet the Global Monitoring Target of a halt in the rise in obesity, regional or local concerted effort is required. Countries will be required to enlist the input of the various governmental and nongovernmental entities essential to the delivery of such a strategy, including those responsible for health, education, food control and standard setting, urban planning, and the environment. With the two main modifiable factors resulting in obesity (diet and physical activity), a multisectoral, aligned response is also required for long-term improvements, for example, in agriculture, trade, industry, and transportation.

With the exception of Kuwait, tobacco smoking rates were at the lower end of the spectrum, and less than half of the rates seen in other Middle Eastern countries, at 45 to 58 percent. However, because these are self-reported data, they are likely to be underestimates, more so in countries such as the GCC states, where non-cigarette tobacco use is frequent. Tobacco use in the Middle East, including the Gulf region, is characterized by a predominantly male smoking population and the reemergence of alternative tobacco such as *shisha* and *midwakh*, especially among youth.[11] The prevalence of alternative forms of smoking has been reported to be increasing in the United Arab Emirates and the entire GCC.[12] *Shisha* use has increased dramatically, and overall in the Middle East, *shisha* smoking far exceeds cigarette smoking by a ratio of 2:1.[13] *Midwakh* and *dokha* use is an emerging issue that is, as yet, a specific problem for the GCC states. The prevalence is reported as high as 25 percent of university students and 12 percent of the general population, with suggestions of earlier age of onset and greater frequency of use per day compared with cigarettes.[14]

Another reason for the low prevalence of tobacco smoking is the low reported rate in females. Male smoking predominates in almost all Arab countries, with a male to female smoking ratio of approximately 10:1.[15] For *shisha* use the imbalance is much lower, at approximately 2:1 for males to females including GCC states.[16] However, with the increase in smoking rates in adolescent females in several Middle Eastern countries such as Lebanon, Iraq, Iran, Syria, and Jordan, there is a risk of higher future rates of smoking among female adults in the GCC states too. This observation warrants specific targeting of prevention measures.

The Global Monitoring Framework target is a 30 percent relative reduction in tobacco use.[17] In order to achieve this target, tobacco cessation initiatives such as MPOWER intervention must tackle locally specific tobacco issues against *shisha* and *midwakh*—including bans and penalties for vendors and parents who allow *shisha* use among children—and urgent local research to better understand how marketing, pricing, and other cigarette-focused tobacco control initiatives can be successful against *shisha* smoking. It should be recognized that relatively little is known about *midwakh* use. Due to its nature, *midwakh / dokha* use is difficult to regulate but threatens to overtake cigarette smoking as the predominant means of tobacco intake for the young Gulf region population. Until recently, tobacco use in the Middle East and the GCC states has predominantly been by males. Future strategies and policies should tackle the growing use of tobacco by adolescents and young females, using international usage comparisons.

Although the OECD framework does not include all chronic disease risk factors, other data substantiate these findings. The GCC Family Health Study and various other unpublished GCC studies reported similarly excessive rates of CVD risk factors in most of the GCC states, with rates of smoking at 16 to 46 percent; hypertension, 15 to 35 percent; dyslipidaemia, 20 to 45 percent; physical inactivity, 80 to 90 percent; diabetes, 12 to 25 percent; and obesity, 40 to 70 percent. The GCC Family Health Study also reflected markedly lower rates of CVD risk factors in Oman compared with the other GCC states.[18]

The predicted burden from such risk factors is alarming. The United States already spends 75 percent of its healthcare budget on chronic disease. Although the average age of the GCC's population is currently approximately two decades younger, aging is predicted to bring with it a tide of chronic disease and financial burden.

CHRONIC DISEASE MORTALITY

CVD mortality rates for all the GCC states, with the exception of Qatar, are already within the top ten countries compared in this study. This is due to a combination of factors. For patients and the public, there is an excess of risk factors, lower public awareness, and lower preventive measures and early detection for CVD and its risk factors in comparison with many of the OECD countries. Hospital factors may also play a role, with lower rates of percutaneous coronary arterioplasty used as a first-line treatment for myocardial infarctions, lower rates of thrombolysis for strokes, and less access to prevention for those with an early onset of symptoms.

The Global Monitoring Target for CVD mortality is a 25 percent relative reduction by 2025.[19] In order to achieve this target in the GCC states, a shift is required from a curative to preventive focus for healthcare, with a change in the healthcare infrastructure to support risk factor management and chronic disease management. Outside the health sector, a multisectoral, joint response is required to align agriculture, trade, industry, and transportation, all of which are essential to promote improved diets and increased physical activity among the population.

Cancer mortality for all the GCC states was less than half the OECD average and at the lowest end of the range of comparison countries. This is likely due to a combination of factors, including the younger age of the population, a more recent onset of the lifestyle change and risk factor burden, lower smoking rates, higher fertility rates (which is relevant for breast cancer), and a likelihood of lower reporting of cancer cases in the region. Cancer registries remain incomplete or nonexistent in the region. Patients from the Gulf region also commonly seek treatment internationally rather than locally for cancer treatment; these cases may remain unrecorded in the existing cancer registries.[20] However, where reliable data are available for cancer incidence—for example, for breast cancer in the United Arab Emirates—the rates are close to the mean for the OECD countries and not in excess, unlike CVD.[21]

The Global Monitoring Framework target for cancer is a 25 percent relative reduction in overall mortality.[22] In order to achieve this target in the GCC, programs for early detection are required—for example, national screening initiatives involving healthcare regulators, payers, and providers, such as call/recall systems and screening databases. To monitor the current status and future changes, better surveillance systems are required, such as national cancer registries.

RELEVANCE OF FINDINGS

The findings of this chapter corroborate data output from Abu Dhabi's health regulator, the Health Authority—Abu Dhabi, in predicting a growth in demand for healthcare services associated with the prevention and treatment of cancer,

CVD, diabetes, respiratory conditions, emergency medicine, and neuropsychiatric conditions.[23] Growth in demand for outpatient services is generally anticipated to be greater than for in-patient services due to the chronic nature of the conditions.

The data from the current study suggest that modifiable, lifestyle-related conditions are on the increase in all the GCC states and are at extremes of prevalence. This, together with aging of this young population, predicts a concomitant sharp increase in required healthcare spending. In addition to increasing healthcare spending, changes in the provision of the type of healthcare will be needed to shift from curative to preventive care, from secondary to primary care, and to more efficient and innovate ways of delivering healthcare. Existing payment models for healthcare services in the GCC states, most of which are based on traditional fee-for-service and bundled/diagnosis-related groups models, will need to accommodate the changes in demand for and the nature of healthcare services.

STRENGTH AND LIMITATIONS

This chapter represents one of the few reports to investigate and compare the chronic disease profiles of the GCC states. It utilizes well-validated, reliable indicators and methodology, including benchmarking against well-described healthcare systems. The OECD framework was found to be the best fit for this study due to its relevance to the known health burden of the GCC states. However, it does not detail all chronic disease indicators; and data to enable comparisons of all the GCC states were not available for several of the OECD framework indicators. The OECD framework does not have indicators for all chronic diseases, such as mental health and musculoskeletal disease. However, some of the main risk factors and the ultimate disease end point of mortality were available for the two main components of chronic disease—namely, CVD and cancer.

THE IMPACT OF THE FINDINGS, AND FUTURE INTERVENTIONS TO ENCOURAGE PREVENTION

The GCC region has an unusual situation, with a high income but relatively poor access to and poor awareness of healthcare. Consequently, successful solutions from elsewhere cannot necessarily be adopted in the region. The Global Monitoring Targets were set to decrease the rates of most risk factors leading to chronic disease. A status quo approach in the systems of the GCC states' healthcare systems will not enable them to reach these targets. Future interventions should consider prevention, healthcare reform, and further research.

Studies are beginning to show a high burden from other chronic conditions in the GCC region, including mental health disorders, musculoskeletal disease, and liver and chronic kidney diseases. Although data remain sparse, these changes can be explained by known changes, such as an increase in the detection and diagnosis of mental health disorders through improved awareness and healthcare provision, the aging of the population and increased obesity leading to greater musculoskeletal disorders and liver disease, and very high rates of diabetes-induced kidney disease. Future screening and monitoring for these conditions is vital.

The prevention of chronic conditions falls both within and outside the health sector. Although there has been great progress in other regions toward a multi-agency approach to tackling the lifestyle factors that lead to chronic disease—such as diet, physical activity, and smoking—any preventive activities in the GCC region have been led solely by the healthcare sector.[24]

Tackling all the known preventive measures is unlikely to enable the GCC states to hit the 2025 targets, for CVD in particular, but it will contribute to the long-term and sustainable change in the next generation. Further momentum is required in establishing preventive programs aimed at children and young adults for the long-term success of such preventive measures.

The Ladder of Interventions used by the UK government is a framework that reports on levels of public health intervention deployed by governments, using the rungs of a ladder as an analogy.[25] The lowest rung represents the status of doing nothing, followed by providing information, enabling choice, guiding choice through changing the default policy, using incentives and disincentives, restricting choice, and, finally, eliminating choice.

In the GCC, most of the public health interventions fall at the second- and third-lowest rungs of providing information and monitoring. In order to achieve change and avoid the status quo, the various stakeholders in the GCC need to move up the ladder of intervention to adopt "healthy default scenarios," to look at the field of behavioral economics in order to guide choice through the use of incentives and disincentives for health, and to restrict choice if necessary. Regional examples include the United Arab Emirates' Weqaya program, which enabled choice, and the restriction of choice of *shisha* smoking in the emirate of Sharjah in the UAE. For those with risk factors for chronic disease, we really need to revolutionize how they interact with the healthcare system (and their lifestyle choices) to avoid a CVD epidemic.

FUNDING THE HEALTHCARE SYSTEM

The health system funding models in the GCC are generally all fee-for-service models, whereby the providers benefit from more activity to help sick patients. There is a disincentive to improve the health of their patients to an extent that keeps them out of hospitals. The GCC should consider moving away from this model as the only payment mechanism for delivering healthcare, especially for chronic disease. Models that reward chronic disease patients being well controlled—for example, disease management programs and payment for quality—are needed. An example is the Quality and Outcomes Framework in the United Kingdom's primary healthcare sector, which rewards general practitioners for better processes for chronic disease (e.g., monitoring, treating, and outcomes such as controlling disease indicators).[26] But to institute this type of payment, there is a need for an "attributable" physician, such as a general practitioner, or a gatekeeping model.

International patient treatment continues to make up approximately 25 percent of all healthcare costs in some of the GCC states, with cancer and rehabilitation cases making up a large proportion of the burden of international care.[27] This reflects the need for improvement in healthcare service provision for these specialties, which would be delivered at much less burden to the country's healthcare budget.

A SHIFT IN THE HEALTHCARE SYSTEM FROM SECONDARY TO PRIMARY CARE

The ideal for the long-term management of chronic disease is a service led by primary care. The GCC states rely heavily on secondary care, however, and have only underdeveloped and underutilized primary care services, with no models to ensure continuity of care through an attributable physician. International examples—such as the patient-centered, home care model in the United States and the vascular checks model in the United Kingdom—aim to provide continuity of care and improved control over chronic disease.

END POINTS FOR THE TREATMENT OF DISEASE

Together with preventing CVD, other disease end points, such as myocardial infarctions and strokes, also warrant further attention, which otherwise will translate into sharp risks for CVD mortality rates during the next two decades. Such preventive measures will be necessary if the GMT goal of 25 percent decrease by 2025 is to be met.[28]

For myocardial infarctions and strokes, international guidelines recommend treatment within a few hours with percutaneous coronary intervention and thrombolysis. In order to deliver this, there is a need for better patient awareness and a stronger healthcare infrastructure—for example, the patient needs to be able to recognize the symptoms and call the ambulance promptly, and the ambulance staff members need to provide a timely response and take the patient to a cardiac facility, where there needs to be an on-site specialist staff (e.g., a cardiologist to deliver the intervention). Thus a system-level change is required.

The secondary prevention of CVD events will become increasingly important as the population ages and the incidence of such events increases. Both physicians' and patients' emphases on secondary prevention remain low compared with Western populations. A study comparing post-myocardial infarction medication use found that at twelve months after the event, only about one-third of patients in the United Arab Emirates were still taking medications, compared with about two-thirds of similar patients in the Swedish Myocardial Infarction Registry.[29]

DEVELOPING CLINICAL RESOURCES BETTER SUITED TO MANAGING CHRONIC DISEASES

The healthcare infrastructure in the GCC states consists of mainstream health sector facilities and personnel and lacks the broader foundation that has developed elsewhere to tackle chronic disease—such as disease management and case management programs; multidisciplinary teams and health support staff, such as health educators; and expanded roles for nursing staff and pharmacists. The healthcare system funding models currently being followed in the GCC region in fact do enable such personnel and infrastructure to develop, but only when the region's funding models change can we expect a broader healthcare system response to the management of chronic disease.

RESEARCH

The epidemiology of the chronic disease burden is better described for CVD but is very poorly described for cancers and mental health issues. Awareness of the disease burden is a preliminary step in being able to tackle the issue at the system level and to develop the necessary resources. Although studies of CVD are now emerging, these are on the whole either small-scale, opportunistic studies or at the emirate level. There are sparse GCC-wide or multisite studies that accurately reflect the chronic disease burden. This work should also form the basis for further research on the drivers of chronic disease in the GCC region.

CONCLUSION

This chapter has sought to quantify the chronic disease burden for the GCC states and to compare them with Western and other benchmark countries. It has found a differential burden of chronic disease with the two main components, with extremes of risk factors and mortality for CVD in most of the GCC states, but much lower cancer mortality.

The chapter has highlighted an approach to next steps in identifying and dealing with the chronic disease burden in the GCC. Future research should also focus on the chronic conditions that are causing significant morbidity in the population—including mental health, musculoskeletal, liver, and kidney disorders—in addition to the financial burden of chronic disease.

NOTES

1. This work was solely conducted by Cother Hajat, who designed the study, conducted the data analysis, and wrote the manuscript. Secondary data only were used for this study. Hajat was adjunct clinical associate professor at the United Arab Emirates University during this time and received no funding for this study. Ali H. Mokdad, Sara Jaber, Muna I. Abdel Aziz, et al., "The State of Health in the Arab World, 1990–2010: An Analysis of the Burden of Diseases, Injuries, and Risk Factors," *The Lancet* 383, no. 9914 (January 2014): 383.

2. For a useful color illustration of this, I recommend seeing the figure from the Institute of Health Metrics and Evaluation at http://ihmeuw.org/3zwc.

3. OECD, "OECD Health Data 2007: Statistics and Indicators for 30 Countries," 2007, www.oecd.org/els/health-systems/health-data.htm.

4. These are WHO data, sourced from the World Obesity Federation, www.worldobesity.org /aboutobesity/world-map-obesity/.

5. OECD, "OECD Health Data 2007."

6. R. Lakhtakia, "Conspicuous Consumption and Sedentary Living: Is This Our Legacy to Our Children?" *Sultan Qaboos University Medical Journal* 13, no. 3 (August 2013): 336–40.

7. International Diabetes Federation, *International Diabetes Federation Atlas, 5th Edition* (Brussels: International Diabetes Federation, 2013), www.idf.org/sites/default/files/da5 /IDF%20Diabetes%20Atlas%205th%20edition.pdf.

8. WHO Global Monitoring Framework, "Set of 9 Voluntary Global NCD Targets for

2025," World Health Organization, www.who.int/nmh/global_monitoring_framework/gmf1 _large.jpg?ua=1.

9. Fatma Al-Maskari , Mohammed El-Sadig, and Nicholas Nagelkerke, "Assessment of the Direct Medical Costs of Diabetes Mellitus and Its Complications in the United Arab Emirates," *BMC Public Health* 10 (2010): 679.

10. WHO data, sourced from the World Obesity Federation, www.worldobesity.org/about obesity/world-map-obesity/.

11. W. Maziak, R. Nakkash, R. Bahelah, A. Husseini, N. Fanous, and T. Eissenberg, "Tobacco in the Arab World: Old and New Epidemics amidst Policy Paralysis," *Health Policy Plan* 6 (2014): 784–94, doi: 10.1093/heapol/czt055.

12. S. Vupputuri, C. Hajat, M. Al-Houqani, et al., "Midwakh/Dokha Tobacco Use in the Middle East: Much to Learn," *Tobacco Control*, 2013, doi: 10.1136/tobaccocontrol-2013 -051530; M. Jayakumary, S. Jayadevan, A. V. Ranade, and E. Mathew, "Prevalence and Pattern of Dokha Use among Medical and Allied Health Students in Ajman, United Arab Emirates,"*Asian Pacific Journal of Cancer Prevention* 11, no. 6 (2010): 1547–49; World Health Organization, "Prevalence of Tobacco Use among Adults and Adolescents," 2009, http:// gamapserver.who.int /gho/interactive_charts/tobacco/use/atlas.html.

13. Maziak et al., "Tobacco in the Arab World."

14. Vupputuri et al., "*Midwakh/Dokha* Tobacco Use"; Jayakumary et al., "Prevalence and Pattern of Dokha Use"; World Health Organization, "Prevalence of Tobacco Use."

15. Maziak et al., "Tobacco in the Arab World."

16. Ibid.

17. WHO Global Monitoring Framework, "Set of 9 Voluntary Global NCD Targets."

18. Tawfik A. Khoja, "Strategic Approaches in Combating Diabetes Mellitus among GCC Countries," 2009, https://view.officeapps.live.com/op/view.aspx?src=http%3A%2F%2Fwww .pitt.edu%2F~super4%2F33011-34001%2F33631.ppt.

19. WHO Global Monitoring Framework.

20. Health Authority Abu Dhabi, "Statistics Manual," www.haad.ae/HAAD/LinkClick.aspx ?fileticket=JY0sMXQXrOU%3d&tabid=349.

21. C. Hajat, J. Taher, W. Sabih, and O. Harrison, "Dramatic Improvements in Breast Cancer Screening Rates in Abu Dhabi, UAE," paper presented at the 15th International Breast Symposium, Cairo, October 2009.

22. WHO Global Monitoring Framework.

23. Health Authority Abu Dhabi, "Statistics Manual."

24. The source for this is a Vitality Institute document.

25. Nuffield Council on Bioethics, "Policy Process and Practice," http://nuffieldbioethics.org /report/public-health-2/policy-process-practice/.

26. Health & Social Information Centre, "Quality and Outcomes Framework," www.hscic .gov.uk/qof.

27. The source for this is an HAAD statistics manual.

28. WHO Global Monitoring Framework.

29. Oliver Harrison, Khaled Aidha Al Jaberi, Eman S. Hassan, Björn Wettermark, Ana-Marija Gjurovic, and Gunnar Engström, "Utilization of Prophylactic Drug Therapy after Acute Myocardial Infarction in Abu Dhabi and Sweden," *Journal of the Saudi Heart Association* 25, no. 2 (2013): 130.

7

LIFESTYLE DISEASES IN THE GULF COOPERATION COUNCIL STATES

Albert B. Lowenfels and Ravinder Mamtani

The discovery of oil in the Gulf region early in the twentieth century, in states now part of the Gulf Cooperation Council (GCC), was a catalyst for dramatic change in the lifestyles of their inhabitants, and consequently, the factors associated with lifestyle diseases. Formerly, the inhabitants of the region led a nomadic life characterized by simple and limited diets, expending larger amounts of energy than the regional populations of today. The lifestyle of the early twentieth century changed dramatically as motor vehicles replaced traditional, animal-based transportation, and as energy-rich diets became easily available. These changes accelerated further in the twenty-first century, and are closely related to the epidemic of diseases that currently threatens the health and well-being of the region's inhabitants.

It is now known that many diseases—including cardiovascular disease, diabetes, many forms of cancer, and strokes—are strongly related to risk factors that can be classified as "modifiable," or related to lifestyle. These diseases account for approximately half the total global burden of disease. Lifestyle factors have been described as "a set of behaviors that reflect an individual's beliefs and values," and may be associated with physical activity, dietary practices, the use of tobacco products, and motor vehicle driving habits.[1] Obesity—a major consequence of negative lifestyle factors—is now more prevalent than malnutrition. And although smoking is on the decline in many countries of the world, it is still a major risk factor in the GCC states.

The states included in the GCC have had a triangular-shaped population pyramid, with high numbers of young people compared with older age groups. In the coming decades, this structure is projected to shift, with the number of older persons—among whom lifestyle diseases are common—increasing relative to the younger population. Consequently, a major effort must be made through-out the region to prevent a potential epidemic of preventable, lifestyle-related illnesses.

How can the impact of lifestyle diseases on the population of the GCC states be measured? The World Health Organization (WHO) reports statistics regard-ing the frequency of disease, mortality rates, and life expectancy. The Global Burden of Disease study has estimated the disability resulting from various dis-eases in different countries and different regions of the world.[2] Individual states, through their ministries of health, will also collect detailed health demographics.

In this chapter we provide an overview of the impact of lifestyle risk factors and associated diseases on the six states in the GCC.

THE GCC STATES

The members of the GCC share several distinguishing characteristics related to the incidence of disease. The populations of the member states differ consider-ably, from 1.8 million in Qatar to 29 million in Saudi Arabia. These states have well-established healthcare systems, all of which rank in the top quartile of the 190 countries evaluated by the WHO, with Oman in the highest position, at eighth in the world.[3] Each country has its own ministry of health with overall responsibility for the nation's health, and these ministries share their ideas and developments in established committees working to solve common problems.

The respective populations of the GCC states are generally young; therefore, the prevalence of lifestyle-related diseases such as cardiovascular disease and cancer will increase as the current population ages. The income levels of citizens are high, implying that financial restrictions will not impede the development of a healthcare system with comprehensive preventive medicine programs. There are benefits to health and general well-being from outdoor recreational activi-ties; but the region's hot, dry climate makes participation a challenge, especially during the summer months.

RISK FACTORS

There are many lifestyle risk factors linked to disease, which can either act inde-pendently of one another or, more frequently, are evident concurrently. These factors commonly include obesity, poor diets, tobacco use, alcohol consump-tion, inadequate exercise, and other, less-well-recognized factors.

A risk analysis focusing on lifestyle factors in relation to the health of the adult population was undertaken for Qatar and Kuwait; in both states, the proportion of the population estimated to have a completely healthy lifestyle (i.e., no major risk factors present) was less than 1 percent, whereas the percentage of the population with three or more risk factors (daily smoking, inadequate diet, decreased physical activity, being overweight, or having an elevated blood pressure) was about 50 percent for Qatar and 75 percent for Kuwait.[4] It is likely that findings for the other GCC states would be similar.

Obesity

Throughout the Middle East, obesity is the most common lifestyle risk factor leading to disease. Body mass index (BMI; i.e., weight in kilograms divided by the square of height, measured in meters) is a widely used measure and is usually preferred to a simple measure of weight alone. Persons with a BMI of 25 to 29.9 are considered overweight, and those whose BMI is equal to or greater than 30 are classified as obese. With the exception of Oman, where obesity rates are lower, the adult obesity rates in GCC states range from 34 to 44 percent in females and 23 to 31 percent in males. These rates were obtained after 2000; more recent 2012 data from Qatar have since revealed that obesity rates in that country have now reached 43 percent in females and 40 percent in males.[5]

Many studies have looked at the relation between obesity and mortality from any cause. A recent study in the United States that monitored nearly one million people for a period of three decades found that all-cause mortality rises steadily with increasing BMI.[6] For those with a BMI greater than 40 (the morbidly obese group), the mortality rate was 250 percent higher than those with a normal BMI. In males there is a strong, nearly linear correlation between BMI and mortality, and similar patterns are exhibited in females. These findings strongly reinforce the recommendation of avoiding obesity throughout a person's lifetime.

In addition to the overall BMI, the distribution of fat within the body is an important risk factor for disease; fat accumulated around the abdomen and waist is more dangerous than fat stored in the hips or thighs. Expressed visually, "apple-shaped" body contours are more of a health risk than "pear-shaped" bodies. In the Middle-East, a high waist-to-hip ratio denoting an apple shape is more common than in Western regions and countries such as Europe, the United States, and Australia.[7]

Diet

In addition to the obesity-causing calorific content of one's diet, nutritional quality is also important for maintaining a healthy lifestyle and reducing the risk of disease. Current recommendations from several health organizations stress the need to consume large quantities of fruit and vegetables, reduce meat consumption, and to substitute whole-grain products for refined carbohydrates. The "Mediterranean diet" captures these recommendations with the addition of nuts and olive oil. Consuming a nutritious diet reduces the overall risk of premature death, and also of death from cancer and cardiovascular disease.[8]

Tobacco Use

In all the GCC states, the prevalence of cigarette smoking is much higher in males than in females, and is higher in younger age groups than older ones. For lifetime smokers, the overall impact on mortality has been extensively studied in many different countries—about half of all smokers will die of smoking-related diseases; and in terms of life expectancy, smokers will lose about ten years of life compared with nonsmokers. Smoking cessation at about the age of thirty years will prevent most of the deleterious effects of this habit.[9]

One form of tobacco use in the GCC states that deserves special mention is the smoking of water pipes, known as *shisha*, which is becoming increasingly popular among teenagers and young adults. In recent studies in Qatar, 22 percent of high school students and 34 percent of college students had used water pipes, ranging from just once to on a regular basis.[10] Water pipe popularity among the young is predominantly driven by the introduction of flavored manufactured tobacco, its availability in cafés, and the lack of regulations specific to water pipe use.

Table 7.1 provides data for the frequency of smoking and obesity in the six GCC states. Tobacco data are derived from 2012 WHO survey data, and obesity data were collected in 2008.[11] Some of the country-specific tobacco and obesity differences may be due to differences in sampling methods or the year of data collection.

Alcohol Consumption

Because of the high proportion of nondrinkers in the population, overall alcohol consumption in the GCC populations is low, accounting for the reduced frequency of alcohol-related diseases in the region. In the combined Middle East and North African region, alcohol and alcohol-related illnesses are ranked thirty-seventh as a cause of disability, compared with a ranking of twelfth in other global regions.

Average alcohol consumption in the Middle-East is about 1 liter of pure

Table 7.1 **The Prevalence of Adult Tobacco Use and Obesity in the GCC States (percent)**

Country	Tobacco Consumption		Obesity	
	Males	Females	Males	Females
Bahrain	31	6	23	34
Kuwait	38	3	34	41
Oman	12	<1	17	24
Qatar	29	<1	31	38
Saudi Arabia	35	6	26	44
United Arab Emirates	18	1	26	40

Sources: World Health Organization, "WHO Report on the Global Tobacco Epidemic, 2015: Bahrain," 2015, http://who.int/tobacco/surveillance/policy/country_profile/bhr.pdf?ua=1; World Health Organization, "Global Database on Body Mass Index," http://apps.who.int/bmi/index.jsp.

alcohol per capita per year, of which about half is believed to be unrecorded consumption—either produced within the region or imported illegally.[12] Despite these low estimates, alcohol consumption by those who do drink is much higher, averaging about 20 liters for males and 11 liters for females, per capita per year. These consumption levels are surprisingly similar to consumption levels for drinkers in non-Muslim countries.[13] Because consumption levels are low on average, there is a relatively low incidence of alcohol-related lifestyle disease in the GCC states. For example, only about 7 percent of motor vehicle injuries in males in the GCC states are believed to be related to alcohol, compared with 19 percent and 33 percent, respectively, in France and Hungary—two countries with relatively high levels of alcohol consumption.

A Sedentary Lifestyle

With the rapid urbanization of the GCC populations, a sedentary lifestyle has become the norm; regional WHO surveys reveal that the majority of the adult population reports less than ten minutes of vigorous exercise per day.

LIFESTYLE-RELATED DISEASES AND INJURIES

Table 7.2 displays the estimated average percentage of years of life lost to lifestyle-related diseases or injuries. From the country-specific profiles of the global burden of disease, more than 25 percent of the burden of disease in the GCC states is caused by lifestyle factors.[14] Control of lifestyle-related diseases in the GCC states would result in a major reduction of illness and death in this region.

Table 7.2 **Percentage of Total Years' Life Lost Attributable to Lifestyle-Related Diseases in the GCC States**

Country	% of Years' Life Lost
Bahrain	31.8
Kuwait	32.8
Oman	19.3
Qatar	21.3
Saudi Arabia	27.5
United Arab Emirates	27.2
Average	26.6

Source: Data from Institute for Health Metrics and Evaluation, "Global Burden of Disease," 2014, https://www.healthdata.org/gbd.

Motor Vehicle Injuries

Across all the GCC states, motor vehicle injuries are the main cause of premature mortality, accounting for about 15 percent of the overall disease burden. Although alcohol consumption is not a major factor in causing these injuries, motor vehicle collisions are often related to aggressive driving and other risk-taking habits that can be avoided. Population attitudes toward risk and risk-taking behavior can be strong factors contributing to motor vehicle injuries. Promoting safe driving through educational programs and driver-training courses, and strict enforcement of existing driving regulations can all play important roles in reducing vehicular-related injuries and deaths in the GCC states.

Circulatory Disease

Cardiovascular disease, hypertension, and strokes account for about 20 percent of all lifestyle-related diseases in the GCC states. Smoking, poor nutrition, and insufficient exercise are the major risk factors for circulatory diseases, and thus all three must be tackled in order to reduce the morbidity and mortality associated with cardiovascular disease. As the regional population ages, the risk of circulatory diseases will increase dramatically.

Diabetes

Diabetes has been described as "the curse of wealth." Since 1990, the frequency of diabetes has increased significantly in all wealthy countries, but especially in the GCC states, where its prevalence is about 15 to 20 percent, about double the global average of 8 percent. Obesity is the main risk factor for diabetes, but smoking also contributes; therefore, the control of smoking is another major goal for diabetes control.

With the exception of the uncommon juvenile type, diabetes is usually considered to be a disease of adults, but evidence is accumulating that even in their early teens, children are now showing evidence of pre-diabetes. Unless pre-diabetes can be diagnosed in these children, they will eventually become adult diabetics. Diabetes is also responsible for the development of other non-communicable diseases, including cancer, circulatory diseases, and eye diseases, all of which increase morbidity and mortality.

Cancer

In the Western countries, the lifetime risk of developing a noncutaneous cancer is about 20 percent, and about half of those who do so will die from their cancer. Smoking, a poor diet, alcohol consumption, and a lack of exercise are all lifestyle factors that can cause cancer, but the burden of smoking-related cancer is particularly critical, with about three-quarters of all lung cancers related to tobacco use.[15] Other cancers linked to smoking include cancers of the mouth, throat, esophagus, kidney, and bladder. According to a recent estimate, about 20 percent of all cancers (males and females combined) are due to smoking.[16] Most of the evidence related to smoking and cancer is focused on cigarette smoking. But in the GCC states, water pipe smoking is popular, and the long-term detrimental health effects are likely to be as significant as cigarette smoking.

Obesity is also a risk factor for cancer. Although the risk of cancer is only slightly increased among overweight individuals compared with those with a healthy BMI, it increases significantly (50 percent) in morbidly obese individuals.[17]

Cancer rates increase rapidly with age, and because of the relatively young age of the populations of the GCC states, cancer rates are lower than in Europe and North America. Nevertheless, there are already several cancers related to smoking and/or obesity that are becoming prevalent in the region, including colorectal, lung, breast, and ovarian cancers. As the population of the region ages, the burden of cancer will increase unless these countries focus immediately on strengthening preventive programs.

THE PREVENTION OF LIFESTYLE-RELATED DISEASES

The prevention of diseases associated with lifestyle risk factors requires a two-pronged approach—from the individual, and also from the central government through health-promotion programs and legislation.

In Singapore a health promotion board oversees all aspects of well-being, from maternal, infant, and child health, through to screening programs for the adult population. China encourages its large and aging population to participate in regular physical activities, often in groups; and in large cities it is common to observe groups of older people performing synchronized exercises.

The GCC states can learn from successful preventive programs in other countries, and a particular focus needs to be given to strengthening regulations to reduce tobacco smoking because it is such a dominant risk factor for lifestyle-related disease.

Is it possible to motivate individuals living in the GCC states to become more responsible for avoiding lifestyle-related health problems? And if so, what approaches will be most effective? It is of far more value to introduce intervention programs early in life rather than later among the adult population. Such health interventions can start even before birth. The fetus benefits from maternal nutritional assessment and risk avoidance, given that obesity during pregnancy leads to gestational diabetes, increasing the subsequent risk of the child developing obesity and diabetes. Smoking during pregnancy decreases birth weight and has an adverse impact on the subsequent health of the baby. Furthermore, breastfeeding has important health benefits for the baby; yet, within the GCC region, only a small proportion of women follow WHO guidelines (i.e., breast-feeding for six months, and continued breastfeeding along with supplemental food for two years). In 2014 the United Arab Emirates passed a law mandating breastfeeding until the baby is two years of age (with some exceptions), though as yet it is uncertain whether this legislative approach will increase breastfeeding rates.

A focus on children and their teachers will be an important component of any prevention strategy in order to influence behaviors starting at a young age. These programs could include

- School-based nutritional educational programs.
- School-based tobacco interdiction programs.
- Daily exercise as part of the school curriculum.
- Providing areas where girls can exercise. Boys already have access to many exercise activities, whereas similar opportunities are limited for girls.
- Banning tobacco sales near schools.
- Promoting increased team sports for all students, where exercise will be part of an enjoyable activity.

For adults, counseling programs aimed at preventing obesity, pre-diabetes, and hypertension—where early recognition and treatment can prevent subsequent life-threatening disease—must be strengthened, as well as measures to encourage regular brisk physical activity to promote cardiovascular, musculoskeletal, and mental health. Encouraging the use of evidence-based, prudent mind–body approaches that diminish stress and improve quality of life is a step in the right direction.

THE EDUCATION OF MEDICAL PRACTITIONERS

Several reports have documented deficiencies in the knowledge of lifestyle medicine among physicians.[18] Incorporating lifestyle medicine curricula and competencies in medical schools is imperative. Lifestyle medicine should also receive a priority in continuing education programs for licensed health practitioners.

The American College of Lifestyle Medicine defines lifestyle medicine as "the evidence-based practice of helping individuals and families adopt and sustain healthy behaviors that affect health and quality of life. Examples of target patient behaviors include, but are not limited to, eliminating tobacco use, improving diet, increasing physical activity, and moderating alcohol consumption."[19]

Lifestyle medicine also "involves the therapeutic use of lifestyle, such as a predominately whole food, plant-based diet, exercise, stress management, tobacco and alcohol cessation, and other non-drug modalities, to prevent, treat, and, more importantly, reverse the lifestyle-related, chronic disease that's all too prevalent."[20]

Providing medical students with knowledge and skills about this form of intervention will enhance their ability to help patients adopt healthier lifestyles, which will reduce premature mortality and improve quality of life. Suggested topics that can be incorporated in curricula include healthy diets and nutrition, physical activity, sleep, stress management, smoking cessation, alcohol consumption, and lifestyle medicine competencies, including leadership, knowledge, assessment, and management skills.[21]

Integrating lifestyle medicine approaches into primary care and chronic disease management clinical programs is pivotal, and every illness visit from a patient should be an opportunity for healthcare professionals to practice lifestyle medicine. Research programs aimed at understanding the causes of and risk factors for lifestyle-related diseases should be a priority; such programs will help identify interventions and programs that are effective and safe in preventing and/or delaying these diseases. Additionally, adequate reimbursement for services related to behavior-driven risk factor reduction will encourage healthcare practitioners to adopt a proactive approach in practicing lifestyle medicine. Evidence shows that these interventions are highly beneficial investments in a nation's healthcare system because they yield positive results by reducing premature mortality, preventing disease, and improving quality of life.

SUMMARY

Lifestyle-related diseases have emerged as a growing threat to the health of the populations of the GCC states. The average life expectancy for native inhabitants of the region is 76.7 years—higher than global life expectancy but lower than the life expectancy for countries with similar income levels. All six GCC states list obesity as the single greatest risk factor for illness because it increases the risk of both malignant and nonmalignant diseases. Although obesity rates are high for both sexes, they are much higher for females, and perhaps are also related to the ready availability of household help and the reduced opportunity for exercise. Together, all the lifestyle-related diseases account for more than a quarter of all premature mortality in the GCC states—more than the estimated premature mortality caused by motor vehicle injuries.

Effective preventive efforts to combat lifestyle-related diseases will require a different strategy than for infectious diseases; it will require the combined efforts of educators, physicians, nurses, nutritionists, health promotion experts, and public health officials. Furthermore, controlling these diseases will require partnerships between health, food and agriculture, urban planning, trade, foreign affairs, education, and other community development sectors. Special circumstances—such as cultural practices, family values, the local climate, and regional lifestyle factors—must be taken into consideration when developing and implementing population-control approaches.

As the population of the GCC region ages, the burden of lifestyle-related diseases will increase dramatically. One estimate suggests that without effective intervention, the annual cost associated with lifestyle-related diseases in the GCC states will rise to $68 billion by 2022.[22] This projection, if accurate, will neutralize any therapeutic medical advances as well as place a serious financial strain on all the GCC states.

NOTES

1. American College of Lifestyle Medicine, website standards page (no longer active), accessed November 24, 2014, www.lifestylemedicine.org.

2. S. S. Lim, T. Vos, A. D. Flaxman, et al., "A Comparative Risk Assessment of Burden of Disease and Injury Attributable to 67 Risk Factors and Risk Factor Clusters in 21 Regions, 1990–2010: A Systematic Analysis for the Global Burden of Disease Study 2010," *Lancet* 380, no. 9859 (2012): 2224–60.

3. World Health Organization, *The World Health Report 200: Health Systems—Improving Performance* (Geneva: World Health Organization, 2000), www.who.int/whr/2000/en/whr00_en.pdf.

4. Al-Anoud Al-Thani, "Qatar STEPS Survey 2012 Fact Sheet," World Health Organization, 2012, www.who.int/chp/steps/Qatar_FactSheet_2012.pdf; Youssef Al-Nesf, "Kuwait STEPS Survey 2006," World Health Organization, 2006, www.who.int/chp/steps/Kuwait_2006_STEPS_FactSheet.pdf.

5. World Health Organization, "Qatar STEPS Survey 2012 Fact Sheet," www.who.int/chp/steps/Qatar_FactSheet_2012.pdf.

6. A. V. Patel, J. S. Hildebrand, and S. M. Gapstur, "Body Mass Index and All-Cause Mortality in a Large Prospective Cohort of White and Black US Adults," *PLoS One* 9, no. 10 (2014): e109153.

7. M. J. O'Donnell, S. L. Chin, S. Rangarajan, et al., "Global and Regional Effects of Potentially Modifiable Risk Factors Associated with Acute Stroke in 32 Countries (INTERSTROKE): A Case-Control Study," *Lancet* 388, no. 10046 (2016): 761–75.

8. J. Reedy, S. M. Krebs-Smith, P. E. Miller, A. D. Liese, L. L. Kahle, Y. Park, and A. F. Subar, "Higher Diet Quality Is Associated with Decreased Risk of All-Cause, Cardiovascular Disease, and Cancer Mortality among Older Adults," *Journal of Nutrition* 144, no. 6 (2014): 881–89.

9. R. Doll, R. Peto, J. Boreham, and I. Sutherland, "Mortality in Relation to Smoking: 50 Years' Observations on Male British Doctors," *British Medical Journal* 328, no. 7455 (2004): 1519.

10. Second International Conference on Waterpipe Smoking Research, Doha, October 25–27, 2014, http://icws.hamad.qa/en/program/27_october/27_october.aspx.

11. World Health Organization, "WHO Report on the Global Tobacco Epidemic, 2015: Bahrain," World Health Organization, 2015, http://who.int/tobacco/surveillance/policy/country_profile/bhr.pdf?ua=1; World Health Organization, "Global Database on Body Mass Index," World Health Organization, http://apps.who.int/bmi/index.jsp.

12. K. D. Shield, M. Rylett, G. Gmel, T. A. Kehoe-Chan, and J. Rehm, "Global Alcohol Exposure Estimates by Country, Territory and Region for 2005: A Contribution to the Comparative Risk Assessment for the 2010 Global Burden of Disease Study," *Addiction* 108, no. 5 (2013): 912–22.

13. World Health Organization, "Global Status Report on Alcohol and Health: 2014," www.who.int/substance_abuse/publications/global_alcohol_report/en/ 2014.

14. Institute for Health Metrics and Evaluation, "Global Burden of Disease," www.healthdata.org/gbd 2014.

15. Doll et al., "Mortality in Relation to Smoking."

16. D. M. Parkin, "Tobacco-Attributable Cancer Burden in the UK in 2010," *British Journal of Cancer* 6, no. 105, Suppl 2 (2011): S6–S13.

17. E. E. Calle, C. Rodriguez, K. Walker-Thurmond, and M. J. Thun, "Overweight, Obesity, and Mortality from Cancer in a Prospectively Studied Cohort of US Adults," *New England Journal of Medicine* 348, no. 17(2003) 1625–38.

18. L. Lianov and M. Johnson, "Physician Competencies for Prescribing Lifestyle Medicine," *Journal of the American Medical Association* 304, no. 2 (2010): 202–3.

19. American College of Lifestyle Medicine, "Core Competencies," 2015, http://lifestylemedicine.org/Core-Competencies.

20. American College of Lifestyle Medicine, "What Is Lifestyle Medicine?" 2015, http://lifestylemedicine.org/What-is-Lifestyle-Medicine.

21. American College of Lifestyle Medicine, "Core Competencies."

22. Booz & Company, "The $68 Billion Challenge: Quantifying and Tackling the Burden of Chronic Diseases in the GCC," Strategy& (PricewaterhouseCoopers), December 5, 2013, www.strategyand.pwc.com/global/home/what-we-think/reports-white-papers/article-display/the-68-billion-dollar-challenge.

CONCLUSION

Ravinder Mamtani, Albert B. Lowenfels, and Sohaila Cheema

The Arab states of the Persian Gulf region have dedicated enormous re-sources to improving healthcare, and over the course of only thirty to forty years, their health profiles have changed dramatically. There has been a marked improvement in health indicators—such as life expectancy, childhood mortality rates, and the incidence of communicable diseases—as well as an evolution of ef-fective public healthcare systems and quality healthcare delivery across the states that belong to the Gulf Cooperation Council (GCC). Several factors will lead to the further improvement of health in the region, including new state-of-the-art tertiary care institutions, the growth of new healthcare education programs, the development of national health strategies tailored to community needs and innovative research initiatives, and increased health awareness. Additional strengthening of individual healthcare systems must continue to focus on dis-ease prevention, reducing mortality and morbidity rates from common diseases, and alleviating pain and suffering among those with chronic conditions.

Although there have been significant improvements within the region, there have also been considerable challenges facing the health of the GCC population. Some of the most critical challenges include the emergence of lifestyle diseases, such as obesity, diabetes, and heart disease; disability and the impaired quality of life associated with adverse mental health conditions; problems associated with chronic pain; disability associated with an aging population; increasing health costs; and a shortage of healthcare workers. Widespread use of tobacco prod-ucts, sedentary lifestyle habits, unhealthy diets, and unresolved stress are also of serious concern and will require coordinated action by policymakers, educators, and the healthcare profession.

Factors that are likely to influence and drive future healthcare changes in the GCC states include rapid advances in medical technology, including an increas-ing reliance on information technology, such as electronic records and tele-health; a focus on self-care; the widespread use of complementary and alternative medicine; an emphasis on patient safety; changing societal values; new government and hospital regulations; global partnerships; interprofessional education; and a multidisciplinary approach to disease management. All these separate pathways present opportunities for improving healthcare but are also formidable challenges.

The uncertainty associated with the unpredictable nature of infectious diseases, as exhibited recently by influenza and viral epidemics (e.g., Zika and Ebola), will continue to challenge scientists and public health professionals, and may strain (and in some instances drain) health resources worldwide. The recent outbreaks of infectious diseases in the Eastern Mediterranean region are of concern and deserve specific mention—polio and meningitis outbreaks have been reported during the hajj pilgrimage in Saudi Arabia and other countries.[1] Controlling such outbreaks will require a concerted public health action.

Although not specifically covered in this book, other pressing issues that have critical implications for healthcare policy, some of which were mentioned just above, also deserve consideration—including the use of new technology, women's health, the health of the migrant population, personalized medicine, and patient-centered care. What follows is a brief discussion of these issues.

Adopting new and proven technological advances to healthcare has the potential to improve therapeutic and diagnostic abilities, but their premature use could be problematic for their accuracy and safety. Because they are often discussed with hyperbole in the popular media, the new health technologies and practices developed in the West are often adopted by other countries without adequate assessment of their evidence base. These technologies promise to deliver improved diagnoses, more effective treatments, and superior patient outcomes. These potential benefits, however, must be weighed against the known challenges of a premature use of technology without full research, an increase in healthcare costs, the appropriateness of the use of technology in a new setting, and the long-term side effects associated with the use of new technology. Thus it is imperative to exercise caution in integrating new technologies into a healthcare system until they are fully assessed from a risk/benefit perspective.

The example of personalized medicine—a new trend in healthcare delivery that has received worldwide attention—illustrates how medical advancements must be grounded in a substantial body of real-world clinical evidence to justify their adoption, not just overly optimistic beliefs about their potential benefits. Personalized medicine aims to match a unique and precise therapeutic regimen to each individual patient and to reduce the risks based on targeted information gathered from genome analyses, biobank data, and personal health information. But Joyner and Paneth caution us about the emerging unrealistic expectations surrounding personalized medicine in their recent article in the *Journal of the American Medical Association*: "Proponents of personalized medicine should consider tempering their narrative of transformative change and instead communicate a more realistic set of expectations to the public."[2] As the GCC states build their research base while actively promoting the growth of knowledge-based communities, they can be vulnerable to potentially unwise and cost-inefficient investments in new Western technologies that promise revolutionary results in an unrealistically short time span.

One other factor that is likely to have an impact on the healthcare industry is an increasing interest in the delivery of patient-centered care, which strengthens the doctor–patient relationship by focusing on treating the patient as an individual person rather than a disease entity. This empathetic and compassionate approach in healthcare is crucial to reducing human pain and suffering. Many research studies have demonstrated that a patient-centered health approach is not only gaining popularity but also crucially results in improved patient outcomes.[3] As the GCC states move to improve and streamline their healthcare systems, investment in programs that foster and nurture patient-centered care will promote health and also make the systems more sustainable. To be effective, this approach requires healthcare providers to be sensitive to the health problems specific to that population.

Women's health is a priority in the GCC states. Globally, women live an average of seventy-two years, as compared with sixty-eight years for men.[4] However, the longevity benefit is often associated with a lower quality of life for women. Gender-based physical and sexual violence, poor access to healthcare services, and sexually transmitted diseases are just a few of the health risks facing the women of today. Additionally, the frequency of several diseases—such as arthritis, fibromyalgia, anxiety, and depression—are higher among women than men.

The life expectancy of women in the GCC states is similar to that of women in other high-income countries. However, there are certain utilization and healthcare trends of public health importance, examples of which are presented here. For example, with respect to choosing a healthcare provider, many women in the GCC states prefer to see female physicians for obstetrical and gynecological care. In the United States and the United Kingdom, conversely, research study results about gender preferences are not quite as consistent.[5] One study reported a tendency for females to seek same-sex physicians for "routine" and "sensitive" visits.[6]

With respect to breast cancer screening, in most high-income countries programs are well established and are largely acceptable to the female population. However, that is not always the case in the GCC states. A national survey conducted in Saudi Arabia, for example, showed that 90 percent of women reported they had never had a mammogram.[7] In contrast, in 2013, 71 percent of US women age fifty to sixty-four years reported having a mammogram within the past two years.[8] Due to poor breast-screening practices and knowledge among the population, many women in the GCC present with advanced stages of breast cancer. Because breast cancer is both the most common and most potentially preventable cancer in women, it is imperative that the GCC countries develop and implement evidence-based national breast-screening and breast cancer awareness programs.

For infant feeding, there is strong evidence that breastfeeding is the best approach—the World Health Organization recommends exclusive breastfeeding for the first six months of an infant's life. Several studies indicate that breastfeeding practices are suboptimal in the GCC countries, with core and optional indicators at much lower levels than desired by the World Health Organization.[9] The current gaps in breastfeeding knowledge, practices, and recommended guidelines highlight opportunities for improvement in national breastfeeding rates.[10]

It is evident from the national health strategies of the GCC states that women and children's health is a priority. During a United Nations meeting in September 2015, the heads of state and government decided on new Sustainable Development Goals. Although all these goals will have an impact on the health and well-being of women and children, Goal 5—to "achieve gender equality and empower all women and girls"—is particularly relevant to this discussion. Governments and countries need to urgently address the specific healthcare needs of women.

Migrant health issues also need to be addressed and integrated into the overall health plans of each GCC nation. This is an especially important issue because in the GCC there are large populations of migrant workers who perform strenuous and physically challenging jobs. Many of the GCC states are paying increasing attention to international viewpoints on the rights of these workers, and also to human rights declarations and the Cairo Declaration on Human Rights in Islam.[11] Where necessary, laws related to occupational safety need to be strengthened, along with the enforcement of existing laws.

It needs to be mentioned that the relationship between migrant workers' risk of injury and/or mortality and these workers' occupations in the GCC states remains largely unexplored. Case control research studies comparing injuries or mortality among migrant and nonmigrant workers may shed light on whether there is a causal link between migrant status and occupational injury.

In addition to workplace injuries, the control of infectious diseases is another important healthcare issue among migrant workers because they often live and work in close proximity to each other, which exacerbates the spread of contagious diseases. Infections such as the Middle East respiratory syndrome can easily spread from one societal group to another, eventually placing everyone at risk.

This book illustrates how, within a few decades, the GCC states have made great progress in closing the gap in healthcare, which formerly separated the countries of the Gulf region from other high-income countries. Previously, these countries may have wisely adopted scientific discoveries and policies developed elsewhere; now, however, we believe that the GCC states are well placed to take the lead both in advancing the scientific understanding of health and disease and in developing evidence-based, globally relevant policies and programs that are culturally appropriate and effective.

NOTES

1. Ali H. Mokdad, Mohammd Hossein Forouzanfar, Farah Daoud, et al., "Health in Times of Uncertainty in the Eastern Mediterranean Region, 1990–2013: A Systematic Analysis for the Global Burden of Disease Study 2013," *The Lancet* 4 (2016): 704–13, www.thelancet.com/pdfs /journals/langlo/PIIS2214-109X(16)30168-1.pdf.

2. Michael J. Joyner and Nigel Paneth, "Seven Questions for Personalized Medicine," *Journal of the American Medical Association* 314, no. 10 (2015): 999–1000.

3. Ronald M. Epstein and Richard L. Street Jr., "The Values and Value of Patient-Centered Care," *Annals of Family Medicine* 9, no. 2 (2011): 100–103; James Rickert, "Patient Centered Care: What It Means and How to Get There," Health Affairs Blog, January 24, 2012, http:// healthaffairs.org/blog/2012/01/24/patient-centered-care-what-it-means-and-how-to-get-there/.

4. World Health Organization, "10 Facts about Women's Health," 2011, www.who.int /features/factfiles/women/en/; United Nations Statistics Division, "The World's Women 2015: Trends and Statistics," http://unstats.un.org/unsd/gender/worldswomen.html.

5. United Nations Statistics Division, "World's Women 2015."

6. A. Makam, C. S. Mallappa Saroja, and G. Edwards, "Do Women Seeking Care from Obstetrician-Gynaecologists Prefer to See a Female or a Male Doctor?" *Archives of Gynecology Obstetrics* 281, no. 3 (2010): 443–47.

7. Charbel El Bcheraoui, Mohammed Basulaiman, Shelley Wilson, et al., "Breast Cancer Screening in Saudi Arabia: Free but Almost No Takers," *PloS ONE* 10, no. 3 (2015).

8. American Cancer Society, "Cancer Prevention & Early Detection Facts & Figures 2015– 2016," (Atlanta: American Cancer Society, 2015), www.cancer.org/acs/groups/content /@research/documents/webcontent/acspc-045101.pdf.

9. Hadia Radwan, "Patterns and Determinants of Breastfeeding and Complementary Feeding Practices of Emirati Mothers in the United Arab Emirates," *BMC Public Health* 13, no. 171 (2013); S. Al-Kohji, H. A. Said, and N. A. Selim, "Breastfeeding Practice and Determinants among Arab Mothers in Qatar," *Saudi Medical Journal* 33, no. 4 (2012): 436–43; Manal Dashti, Jane A. Scott, Christine A. Edwards, and Mona Al-Sughayer, "Predictors of Breastfeeding Duration among Women in Kuwait: Results of a Prospective Cohort Study," *Nutrients* 6, no. 2 (2014): 711–28.

10. Emma Graham-Harrison, "UAE Law Requires Mothers to Breastfeed for First Two Years," *The Guardian*, February 7, 2014, www.theguardian.com/world/2014/feb/07/uae-law -mothers-breastfeed-first-two-years; Zoi Constantine, "UAE Mothers Divided over Breast-feeding Law," *Al Jazeera*, April 22, 2014, www.aljazeera.com/news/middleeast/2014/04/uae -mothers-divided-over-breastfeeding-law-2014414103843773674.html.

11. Maria Kristiansen and Aziz Sheikh, "The Health of Low-Income Migrant Workers in Gulf Cooperation Council Countries," *Health and Human Rights Journal*, 2014, www.hhr journal.org/2014/07/the-health-of-low-income-migrant-workers-in-gulf-cooperation-council -countries/.

CONTRIBUTORS

SAMIR AL-ADAWI is a professor of behavioral medicine at the College of Medicine of Sultan Qaboos University, and the editor of the *Journal of Scientific Research: Medical Sciences*. His clinical and research interests focus on functional recovery following brain damage and how stress and distress manifest in different populations and cultures. He received his doctorate from the Institute of Psychiatry at King's College London. His selected publications include articles in the *Journal of Autism and Developmental Disorders*, *Child and Adolescent Psychiatry and Mental Health*, and Sultan Qaboos University's *Journal for Scientific Research: Medical Sciences*.

MOHAMAD ALAMEDDINE is an assistant professor in the Department of Health Management and Policy at the American University of Beirut. Previously, he was as a senior research associate and director of international development at the University of Toronto. His research interests include studying health, human resources, labor force dynamics, recruitment and retention practices, and the quality of work environments. He has published papers in multiple journals on health workforce dynamics, especially on the nursing workforces in Lebanon and Canada. He received a PhD in health management and policy from the University of Toronto, and a master's degree in public health from the American University of Beirut.

HASSEN AL-AMIN is an associate professor of psychiatry at Weill Cornell Medicine–Qatar and a consultant to Hamad Medical Corporation. He also serves as the associate director of Weill Cornell's psychiatry clerkship program. His current research interests include several projects related to the translation and cultural adaptation of clinical psychiatric scales to Arab populations.

SOHAILA CHEEMA, MBBS, MPH, is the director of the Division of Global and Public Health and an assistant professor of healthcare policy and research at Weill Cornell Medicine–Qatar. She actively participates in the oversight and implementation of global and public health education, research, and community programs. She is committed to improving the quality of education, and takes pride in teaching public health and related disciplines to premedical and medical students, and also to residents in community medicine. Her research interests are multidisciplinary, with an emphasis on the noncommunicable disease paradigm, particularly in the areas of obesity, diabetes, and road traffic injuries.

SUHAILA GHULOUM is a senior head consultant psychiatrist at Hamad Medical Corporation in Qatar. She is also an assistant professor at Weill Cornell Medicine–Qatar. Her selected publications include "Gender Differences in the Knowledge, Attitude, and Practice towards Mental Health Illness in a Rapidly Developing Arab Society," in the *International Journal of Social Psychiatry* (2011); and "Epidemiological Survey of Knowledge, Attitudes, and Health Literacy concerning Mental Illness," in the *Journal of Primary Care and Community Health* (2010). She received her MD from the Royal College of Surgeons in Ireland and is a member of the Royal College of Psychiatrists in Britain.

COTHER HAJAT is chair of prevention for the Emirates Cardiac Society, adjunct clinical associate professor at the Public Health Institute of the United Arab Emirates University, and a public health adviser. She previously worked for the Health Authority of Abu Dhabi, where she established data-driven programs for cardiovascular disease prevention, breast cancer screening, and smoking cessation. In Britain, she is a fellow of the Faculty of Public Health and a member of the Royal College of Physicians. She has published papers on topics such as cardiovascular screening and tobacco smoking. She received an MPH and a PhD in cardiovascular epidemiology from King's College London.

NOUR KIK is policy and advocacy officer at the National Mental Health Programme of the Ministry of Public Health in Lebanon. She was a member of the drafting and revision team of the Mental Health and Substance Use Prevention, Promotion, and Treatment Strategy for Lebanon 2015–2020, which was launched in May 2015. She coauthored the interventions mapping exercise report *The "4Ws" in Lebanon: Who's Doing What, Where, and until When in Mental Health and Psychosocial Support* (April 2015); and the policy document *Protecting Health Workers from Exposure to Occupational Violence* (January 2015).

NABIL M. KRONFOL is president of the Lebanese Healthcare Management Association and cofounder of the Center for Studies on Aging. He is a retired professor of health policy and management at the American University of Beirut. He is a frequent consultant to the World Health Organization, the World Bank,

UNICEF, and the United Nations Development Program on health systems, human resources, quality assurance, and the health of the elderly. His selected publications include "Public Health, the Medical Profession, and State-Building: A Historical Perspective," in *Public Health in the Arab World*; and "Changing Demographics in the MENA Region: The Need for Social Policies to Drive Opportunities," in *Population Dynamics in Muslim Countries*.

ALBERT B. LOWENFELS, MD, is a professor of surgery and a professor of community and preventive medicine at New York Medical College. He has also served as visiting fellow at the International Agency for Research on Cancer, as a consultant to the US Food and Drug Administration, as a consultant to the International Prevention Research Institute, as a senior investigator for the European Institute of Oncology, and as an external adviser to the grant for genes related to pancreatic cancer funded by the US National Institutes of Health. His research interests, as reflected in more than two hundred publications, include lifestyle diseases, cystic fibrosis, and cancer. He has also contributed to research initiatives on traffic injuries, diabetes, and obesity in Qatar.

RAVINDER MAMTANI, MD, is a professor of healthcare policy and research, and senior associate dean for population health and capacity building at Weill Cornell Medicine Qatar. He is a specialist in occupational and general preventive medicine, public health, and integrative medicine. He previously worked at New York Medical College / Westchester Medical Center, Valhalla. His overall interests include developing innovative education programs, chronic disease management, lifestyle medicine, and integrative health. His research interests include obesity, diabetes, traffic injuries, integrative medicine, and health policy. He is a member of the New York State Board for Professional Medical Conduct.

DIONYSIS MARKAKIS is a lecturer in international relations at Queen Mary University of London. Previously, he was a research associate of the Center for International and Regional Studies at Georgetown University in Qatar. He received a PhD from the London School of Economics and Political Science. His most recent book is *US Democracy Promotion in the Middle East: The Pursuit of Hegemony* (Routledge, 2015).

YARA MOURAD is the program coordinator for the Refugee Research and Policy in the Arab World Program of the Issam Fares Institute for Public Policy and International Affairs at the American University of Beirut. Before joining the Issam Fares Institute, she was a research associate in the Department of Health Management and Policy of the Faculty of Health Sciences at the American University of Beirut, from which she received a BS in nutrition and dietetics and an MS in public health.

RAMI YASSOUB is the health information and data-collection supervisor for Qatar's Supreme Council of Health. His research interests and professional efforts focus on examining public health initiatives that promote population health and coverage through advances in knowledge-transfer capacities. He received a master's degree in public health from the American University of Beirut.

INDEX

Tables and Figures are denoted by *t* and *f* following the page number.

CPSIA information can be obtained
at www.ICGtesting.com
Printed in the USA
FSOW04n1723221017
40071FS